MEDICINE AND BOTANY

An Australian Cadaster

Australian flora named after those whose lives have served medicine and health.

John Hemsley Pearn

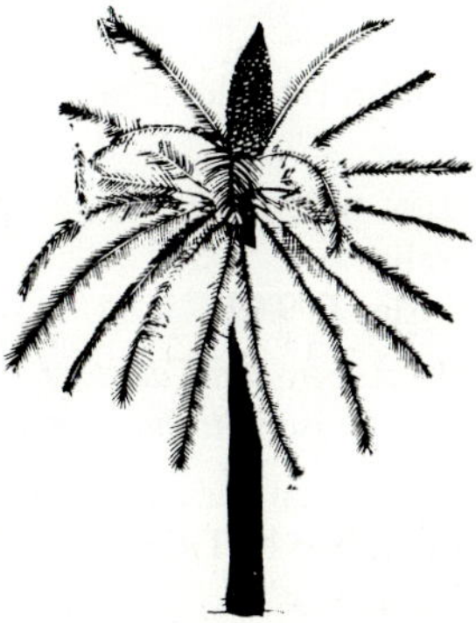

Amphion Press

MEDICINE AND BOTANY
An Australian Cadaster

Bibliography
Illustrations
Includes Index

1st Edition (English)
First published – 1990

Typeset and Published by: Amphion Press, (Department of Child Health Publishing Unit), Department of Child Health, University of Queensland, Royal Children's Hospital, Brisbane, Q. 4029 Australia.

Printed by. Merino Lithographics, 18 Baldock Street, Moorooka, Brisbane, Queensland, 4105, Australia.

Cover by. Robert Allen and Paul Ramsden, The Queensland Museum.

CATALOGUING IN PUBLICATION DATA
National Library of Australia
Author: Pearn, John Hemsley (1940-)
Medicine and Botany – An Australian Cadaster
Australian flora named after those who have served medicine and health.
1. Botany – Australia – Nomenclature. 2. Medicine – Australia – Biography.
3. Medical botanists – Australia. I. Title.
581.994
NATIONAL LIBRARY OF AUSTRALIA CARD NUMBER AND ISBN
ISBN 0 86776 358 2

CONTENTS

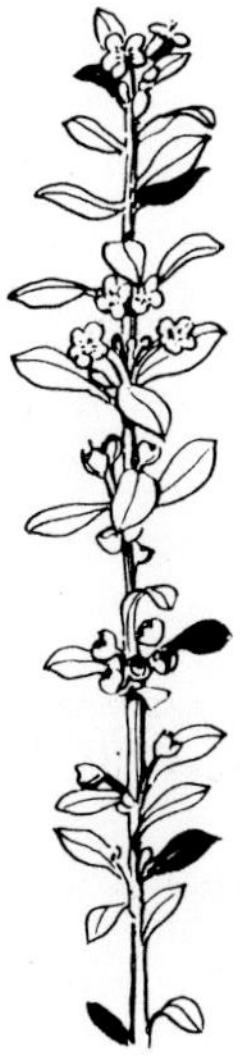

THE COVER

The cover portrays the ground orchid Acianthus ledwardii, recreated by Mr Robert Allen, Artist, of the Queensland Museum, using early specimen illustrations. This orchid occurred in South East Queensland and Northern New South Wales, but is now almost certainly extinct. It commemorates Dr Colin Ledward (1903–1963), a general practitioner and botanist of Canungra, Cloncurry and Burleigh Heads.

SI MONUMENTUM REQUIRIS, CIRCUMSPICE

You'll need no plaque or marble now. You saw
your corner of all future autumns claimed
in Eaglehawk that afternoon your name
was written down a dahlia stake. In time
that still has far to come the people drawn
down aisles of numbered blooms may find
their eyes arrested where the lights that lie
in petals edgings blur
and merge with burgundy. They'll pause,
perhaps, and check their catalogues again.
And read your name.
And wonder who you were.

Mr Frank McMahon
Some Future Festival

From the Anthology *The Asphalt and the Stars*.
Lines written to commemorate the National Dahlia Festival,
held annually at Eaglehawk, Victoria, Australia.

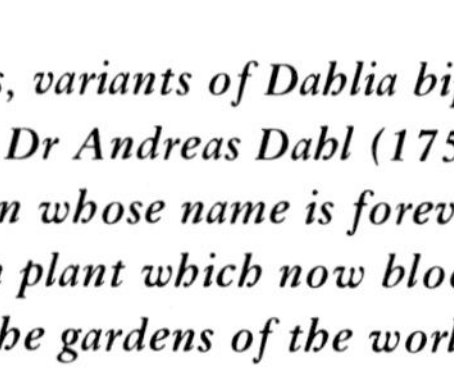

Dahlias, variants of Dahlia bipinnata, named after Dr Andreas Dahl (1751–1789) the Swedish physician whose name is forever commemorated in the Mexican plant which now blooms throughout the gardens of the world.

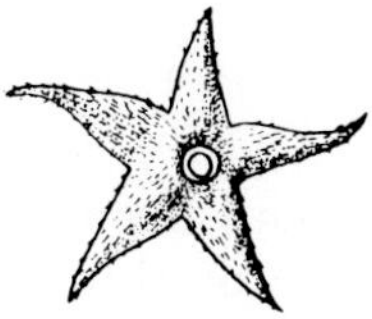

FOREWORD

The histories of medicine and botany have long been intertwined. From earliest recorded history, plants have played a major role in the healing of the ills of all humankind. The early physicians were among the first to study plants in a scientific way; the Greek physician Dioscorides was one of the earliest authorities on plants and plant names, through his interest in medicinal plants. With the development of the University system, teaching about plants was undertaken in medical schools. So it is perhaps not unusual that the father of modern botany, Linnaeus, was sent to a medical school to gain an education and further his childhood interest in plants; and was eventually elevated to the position of Professor of Medicine. In the last two centuries science has become fragmented. Each of its disciplines has built up such a body of specialized information that botany, like its sister sciences, is recognized in its own right. The generalist philosophers, who could be eminent in a broad range of disciplines, are now rarities.

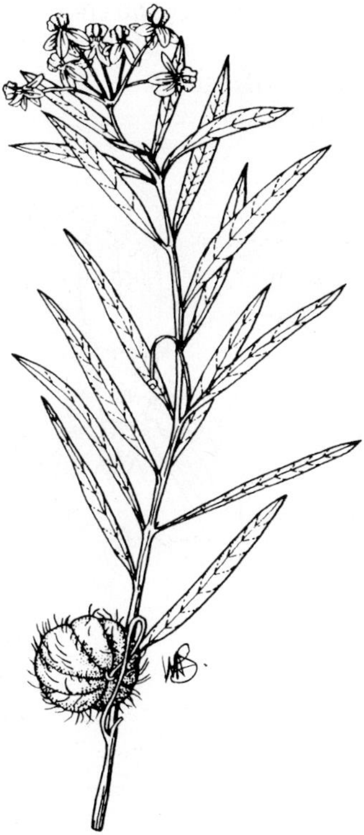

Botanists, like explorers, have recognized their patrons by naming plants after them. The names of benefactors and those who have assisted them in their studies are enshrined in the catalogues of plants in every part of the world. Plant names provide memorials to thousands of people who in some way have helped in the accumulation of knowledge that forms the basis of the history of botany. It is therefore not unusual that medical practitioners have figured prominently in catalogues of plant names.

Foreword

Enthusiasm is contagious and I have admired and been caught up with the enthusiasm John Pearn has shown for this subject. His love of things medical abounds and his scientist's enjoyment of discovery cannot be suppressed. He has tackled the rather daunting task of assembling this information with passion.

Of particular convenience is the index which gives both botanical and common names. A perusal of this index list gives one some perspective of the importance of medicine and its practitioners in the history of Australian botany. It is a living history as the garden and forest thus speak an extra language, that of the lives of doctors here commemorated. Besides being a well researched compendium of information this book is a reminder of the long association of the medical and botanical professions.

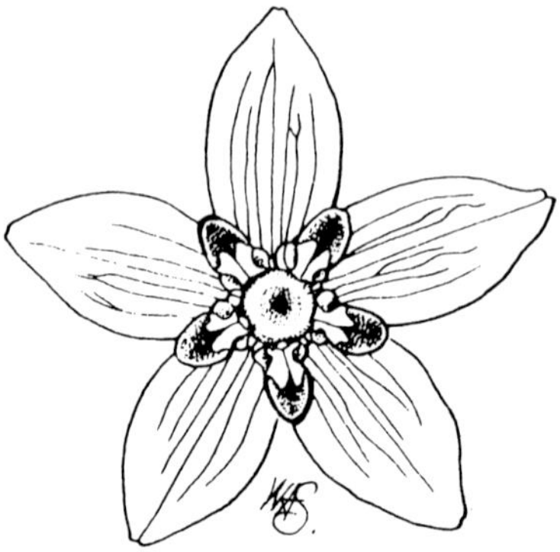

Dr Robert Johnson

Director
The Queensland Herbarium
Brisbane, Australia.

This work was made possible by the generous support and sponsorship of GLAXO AUSTRALIA AND DUNCAN FLOCKHART (QUEENSLAND DIVISION). The author extends special thanks to Mr Ian Munro of Glaxo Australia for his support and encouragement.

PREFACE

Cadaster: A Register of Property, Ownership, and Values, for subsequent call to account.

The annual bloom of a flower is a memorial to the individual after whom it has been named. The repository of scientific names of Australian flora contains much that is relevant to the history of medicine. Indeed, in the Australian bush are to be found the memorials, often the only memorials, of many doctors who have practised their healing art since the earliest times of recorded history.

The Greek physicians, Aesculapius and Euphorbus, are there, as are the Roman doctors who followed them. Galen and Musa could not have imagined the plants that now bear their names, commemorating their lives across a world they could not have imagined, and spanning two millennia of recorded history. The Persian physician, Avicenna, has a living memorial on the seacoasts of Australia. Doctors from Scotland and Switzerland, Romania and Russia, and from Finland and France have their living epitaphs also – in some cases now the only material thing to commemorate their lives – in the Australian flora, which bears their name.

This register of Australian native herbs, shrubs, trees, and aquatic plants records those doctors whose colleagues and successors have immortalized them by incorporating their names in the literature of scientific botany. Thus are the histories of medicine and botany intertwined.

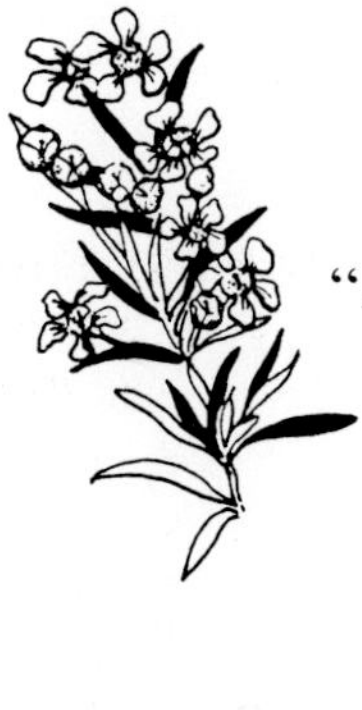

Monumentum aere perennius

"A monument more lasting than bronze"

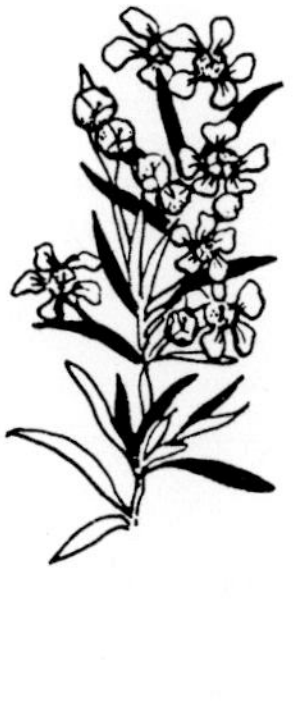

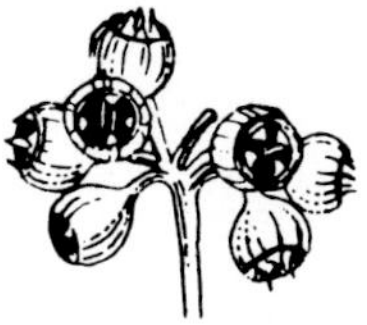

KEY

The primary reference for inclusion in this botanical cadaster is that the plant is a native of Australia, or is an introduced species now established in the wild, or is a specific Australian-bred hybrid.

The list cannot be a definitive or static one, and will expand as new plants are discovered, and as new blooms are bred. The criteria for inclusion of individuals so honoured is that they have primary medical qualifications, or a major life's contribution to the practice of medicine or the maintenance of health. Pharmacists, dentists, nurses and other professional groups are not primarily included, except insofar as their life's work has included major medical themes. An historical compilation of the botanical records of this latter group of health professionals is a task for the future. Several apothecaries have been included in this list, healers whose professional lives were such that they acted as surgeons or physicians, or who made major contributions to the science of medicine and healing.

Many individual doctors have had many different plants named after them. All genera which commemorate an individual are included in this list, and in such cases individual species are not listed. The taxonomic suffix "spp." refers to such instances. In the case of species, one representative species name only is included, although in many instances a single doctor may be commemorated by multiple species, each in a different genus.

Many of the doctors so honoured have made major contributions to science, the arts, and to civic life, in addition to their roles as surgeons, or medical practitioners. Their principal contributions to other non-medical themes in society are also listed.

I have also listed the country or countries in which individuals spent significant parts of their lives. The modern names of countries and regions are listed, and not the original names contemporaneous with the doctor-botanist's life. The traditions of medicine, like the world of plants know no political or national boundaries.

JHP.

ACHILLES, (Trojan War, Greek Mythology) (*c.* 1400–*c.* 1100 B.C.)

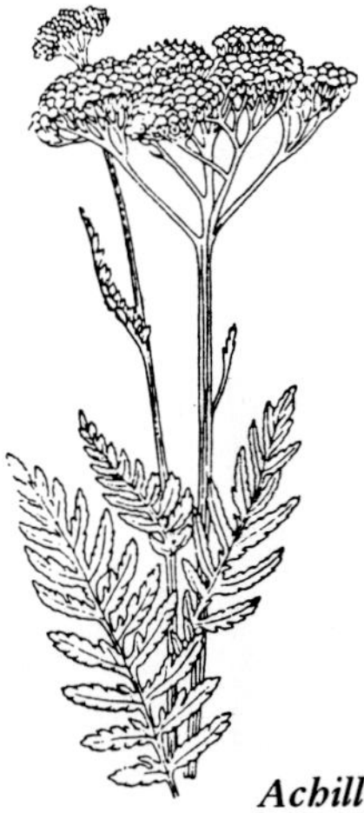

Achillea sp.

Major contributions to medicine, exploration, scholarship and civic life –

Warrior, First Aider

Country of residence and civic and scientific contribution –

Greece (Troy, now Asia Minor)

Scientific Names –

Achillea spp. (An introduced genus, native in Europe, now naturalized in southern Australia.)
Pithocarpa achilleoides

ACKLAND, Dr Thomas (born 1908)

Major contributions to medicine, exploration, scholarship and civic life –

Surgeon

Country of residence and civic and scientific contribution –

Australia (Melbourne)

Scientific Name –

Dahlia bipinnata "Thomas Ackland"

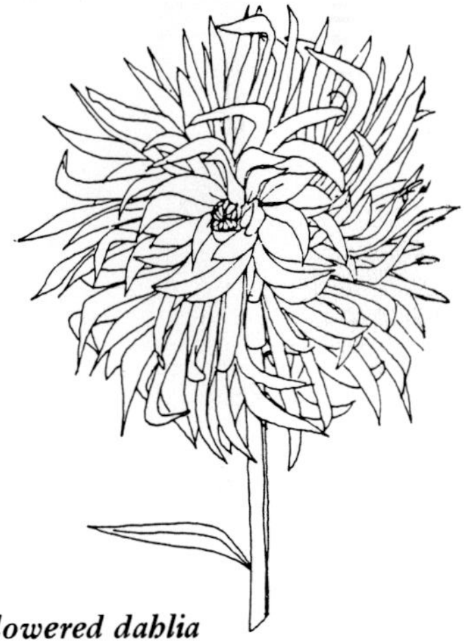

Cactus-flowered dahlia

AFZELIUS, Professor Adam (1750–1837)

Major contributions to medicine, exploration, scholarship and civic life –

Doctor, Botanist

Countries of residence and civic and scientific contribution –

Sweden (Uppsala), West Africa (Sierra Leone), England (London), Scotland

Scientific Name – *Afzelia australis* (syn: *Intsia bijuga*)

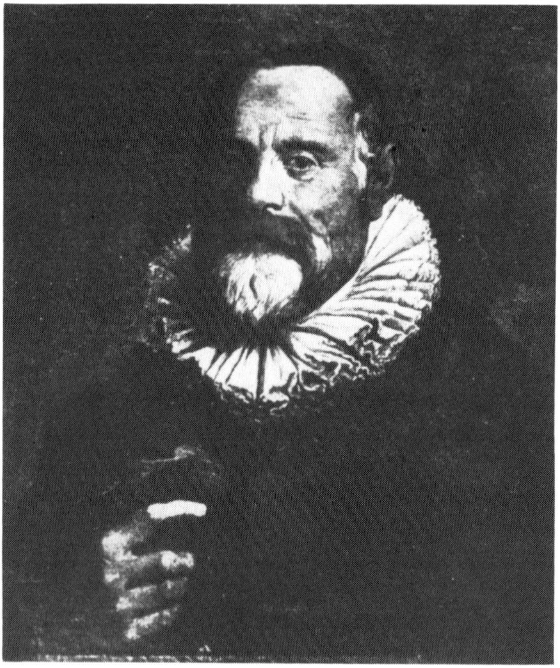

PROFESSOR DOTTORE ULISSE ALDROVANDI (1522–1605)
whose name is commemorated in Aldrovanda versiculosa, the Waterwheel Plant, which traps and digests tiny aquatic life forms in Australian swamps.

ALDROVANDI, Professor Ulisse (1522–1605)

Major contributions to medicine, exploration, scholarship and civic life –

Doctor, Botanist, Zoologist, Anatomist, Embryologist, Writer

Country of residence and civic and scientific contribution –

Italy (Bologna and Padua)

Scientific Name – *Aldrovanda vesiculosa* (a monotypic genus)

ALFRED, Prince (HRH Duke of Edinburgh) (1844–1900)

Major contributions to medicine, exploration, scholarship and civic life –

Sailor, Medical Patron

Countries of residence and civic and scientific contribution –

United Kingdom (London),
Australia (Sydney)

Scientific Name – *Livistona alfredii*

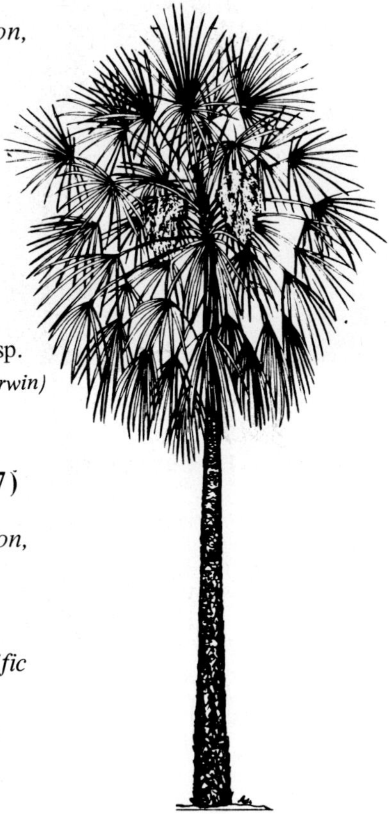

Livistona sp.
(Courtesy of Adi Dunlop, Darwin)

ALPINI, Professor Prosper (1553–1617)

Major contributions to medicine, exploration, scholarship and civic life –

Doctor, Botanist, Economic Botanist

Countries of residence and civic and scientific contribution –

Italy (Venice, Genoa and Padua), Egypt

Scientific Name – *Alpinia* spp.

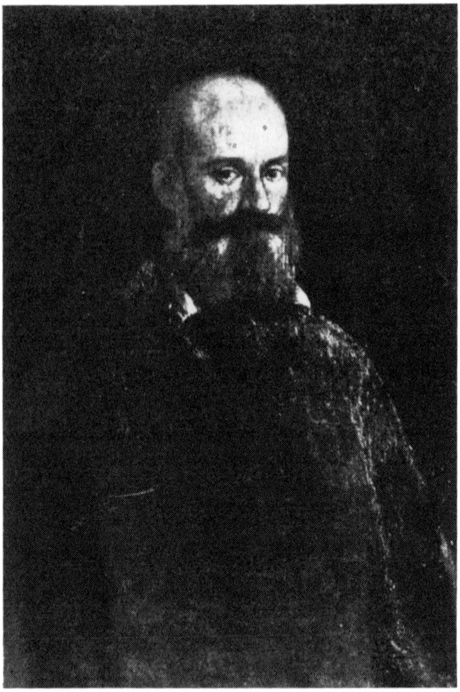

PROFESSOR PROSPER ALPINI
(1553–1617)

Doctor and Botanist of Venice, Genoa and Padua. He travelled and practised in Egypt, and has given his name to several species of wild ginger (eg. Alpinia coerulea) in the rain forests of Northern Australia.

ALSTON, Dr Charles (1685–1760)

Major contributions to medicine, exploration, scholarship and civic life –

Physician, Botanist

Countries of residence and civic and scientific contribution –

England (London), Holland, Scotland (Edinburgh)

Scientific Name – Alstonia spp.

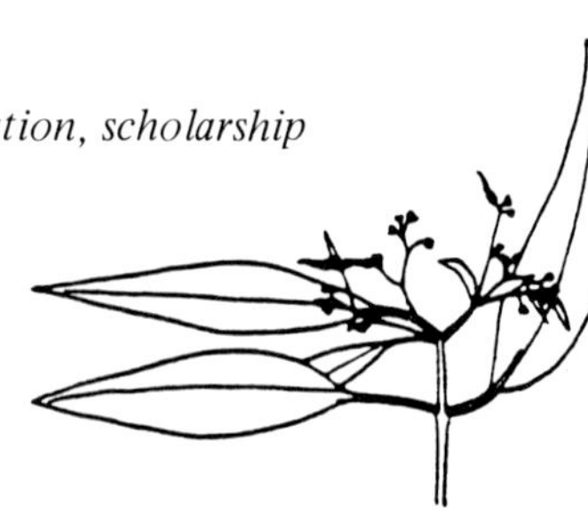

Alstonia constricta

AMMANN, Dr Paul (1634–1691)

Major contributions to medicine, exploration, scholarship and civic life –

Doctor, Botanist

Country of residence and civic and scientific contribution –

Germany (Leipzig)

Scientific Names –

Ammannia spp.
Bergia ammannioides

ANDERSON, Surgeon William (*c.* 1750–1778)

Major contributions to medicine, exploration, scholarship and civic life –

Naval Surgeon, Botanist, Ornithologist

Countries of residence and civic and scientific contribution –

England (North Berwick), Scotland (Edinburgh), Africa, Australia, South America, South Pacific, Antarctica

Scientific Names –

Andersonia spp.
Sprengelia andersonii

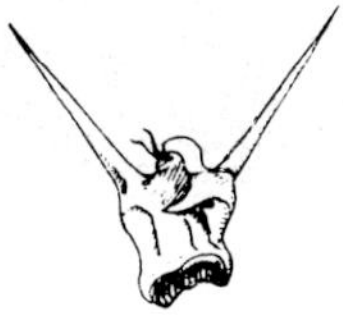

Sclerolaena (syn. ***Bassia***) ***andersonii***

ANGUILLARA, Professor Luigi (1512–1570)

Major contributions to medicine, exploration, scholarship and civic life –

Apothecary, Doctor, Botanist

Country of residence and civic and scientific contribution –

Italy (Bologna, Pisa, Padua, Florence)

Scientific Name – Anguillaria spp.

APJOHN, Professor James (1796–1886)

Major contributions to medicine, exploration, scholarship and civic life –

Doctor, Physical Chemist, Geologist

Country of residence and civic and scientific contribution –

Ireland (Dublin)

Scientific Name – Apjohnia laetevirens

ARISTOTLE (384 B.C. – 322 B.C.)

Major contributions to medicine, exploration, scholarship and civic life –

Philosopher, Natural Historian, Doctor

Country of residence and civic and scientific contribution –

Greece (Athens, Pella, Chalkis)

Scientific Name – Aristotelia spp.

ARNOLD, Surgeon Joseph (1782–1818)

Major contributions to medicine, exploration, scholarship and civic life –

Naval Surgeon, Botanist

Countries of residence and civic and scientific contribution –

England (Suffolk), Scotland (Edinburgh),
Australia, Indonesia, South America

Scientific Name – Arnoldia spp. (syn. *Weinmannia*)

AESCULAPIUS,
THE GOD OF MEDICINE,
with his caduceus,
the staff with entwined serpent of healing.

Beside him stands his daughter,
HYGIEIA,
the Goddess of Health.

(Photo, courtesy of the Vatican Museum, Rome.)

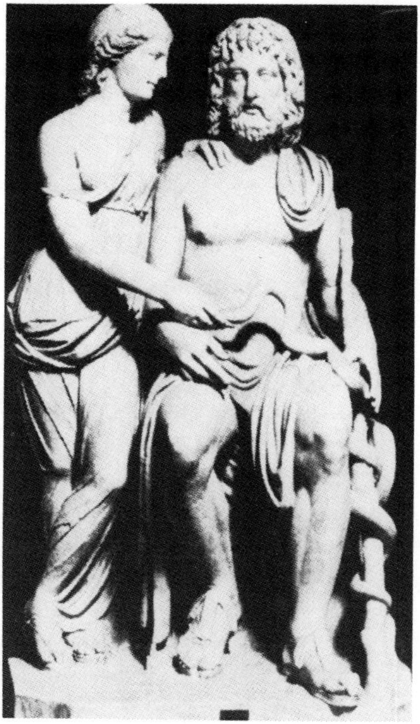

ASCULAPIUS (prior or 600 B.C.)

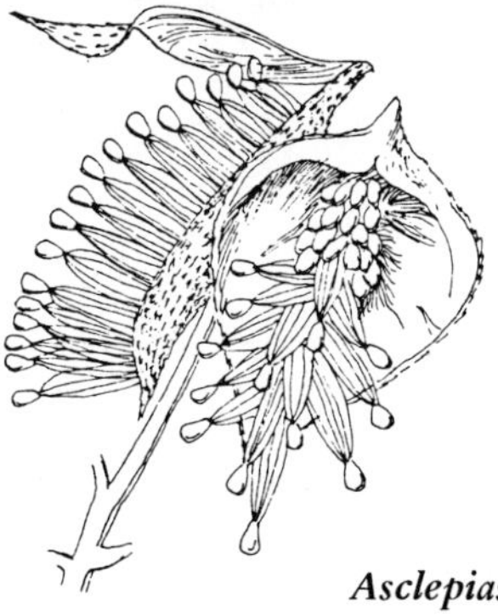

Asclepias sp.

Major contributions to medicine, exploration, scholarship and civic life –

Physician, God of Medicine

Country of residence and civic and scientific contribution –

Greece

Scientific Name – *Asclepias* spp.

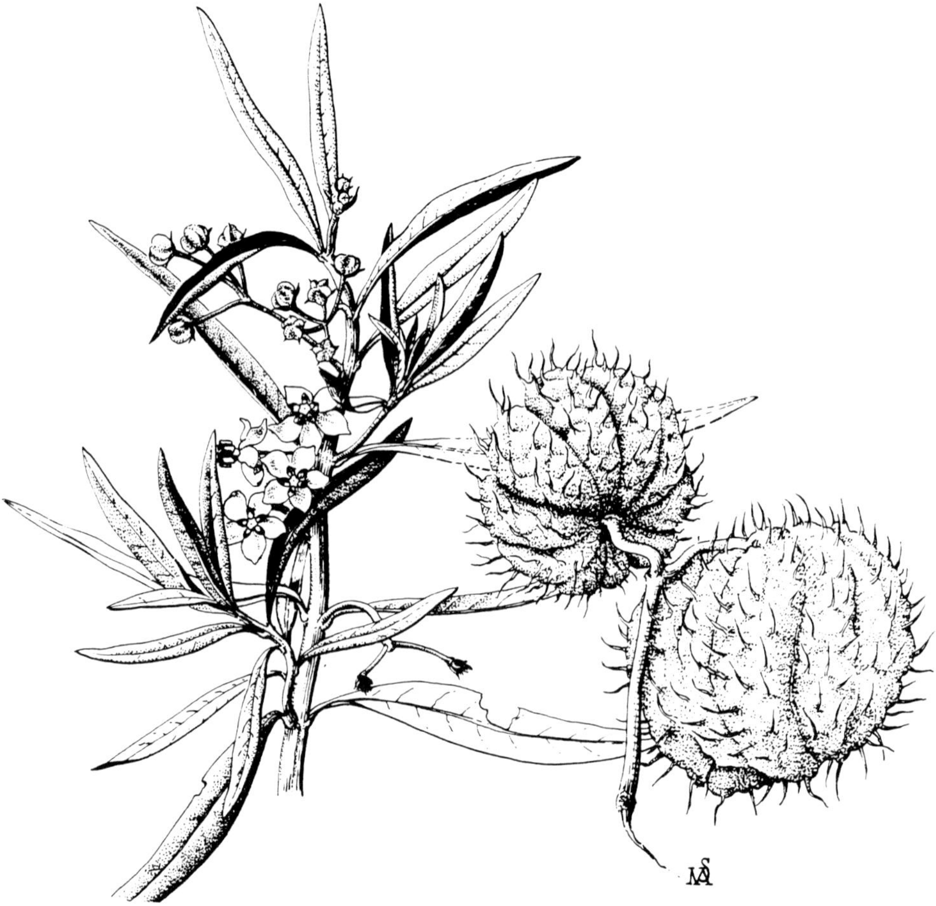

Asclepias physocarpa

"Wild Cotton" from Tamborine Mountain, Queensland.
Asculapius is the legendary western God of Medicine.

Drawing by Margaret Saul, formerly of the Queensland Herbarium.

AVICENNA (980 – 1037)

Major contributions to medicine, exploration, scholarship and civic life –

Physician

Country of residence and civic and scientific contribution –

Persia (now Bokhara, Hamadan, Iran)

Scientific Names –

Avicennia spp.
Abutilon avicennae

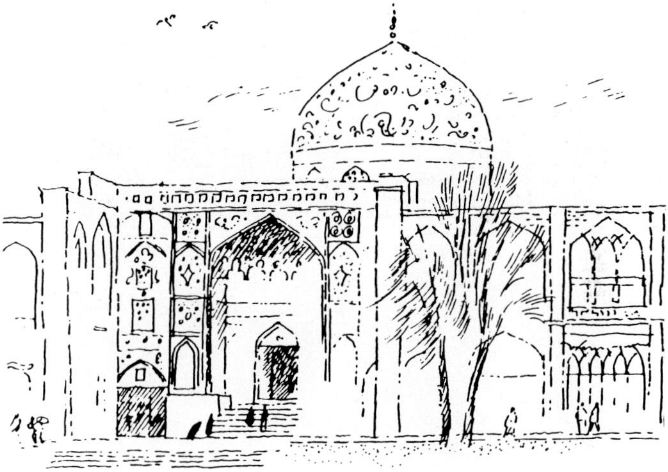

The Arabian influence on Western Medicine and Botany was considerable, primarily through the writing and influence of the physician-botanist Avicenna.

The Australian genus of mangroves, Avicennia, commemorates his name.

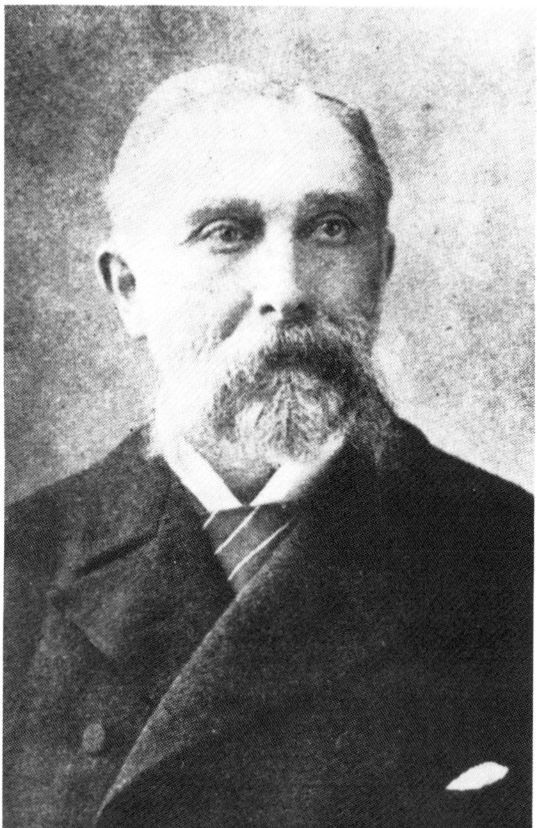

Dr WALTER BALLS-HEADLEY (1841–1919)
of Melbourne,
pioneer obstetrician and gynaecologist in Australia.

Photo courtesy of 'Alma Mater' (1898),
University of Melbourne.

BAECK, Dr Abraham (1713–1795)

Major contributions to medicine, exploration, scholarship and civic life –

Physician, President – Swedish College of Medicine, Botanist

Country of residence and civic and scientific contribution –

Sweden (Uppsala, Stockholm)

Scientific Name – Baeckea spp.

BALLS-HEADLEY, Dr Walter (1841–1919)

Major contributions to medicine, exploration, scholarship and civic life –

Obstetrician, Paediatrician, Surgeon, Writer, University Teacher

Countries of residence and civic and scientific contribution –

England (London, Bideford), Palestine, Australia (Warwick, Melbourne)

Scientific Name – Medinilla balls-headleyi
(This single species only in Australia, of this large genus)

BALOGH, Dr Joseph (*fl.* 1779)

Major contributions to medicine, exploration, scholarship and civic life –

Physician, Botanist

Countries of residence and civic and scientific contribution –

Transylvania (Hungary), and after 1918, Romania, Holland (Leiden), Surinam

Scientific Name – Baloghia spp.

BANCROFT, Dr Joseph (1836–1894)

Major contributions to medicine, exploration, scholarship and civic life –

Physician, Surgeon, Natural Historian, Scientist

Countries of residence and civic and scientific contribution –

England (Cheshire, Nottingham), Australia (Brisbane)

Scientific Names –

Beilschmiedia bancroftii
Elaeocarpus bancroftii

BANCROFT, Dr Thomas Lane (1860–1933)

Major contributions to medicine, exploration, scholarship and civic life –

Doctor, Botanist, Zoologist

Country of residence and civic and scientific contribution –

Australia (Brisbane, Innisfail, Deception Bay, Stannary Hills [near Cairns], Eidsvold)

Scientific Names –

Sarcochilus bancroftii
Strychnos bancroftiana

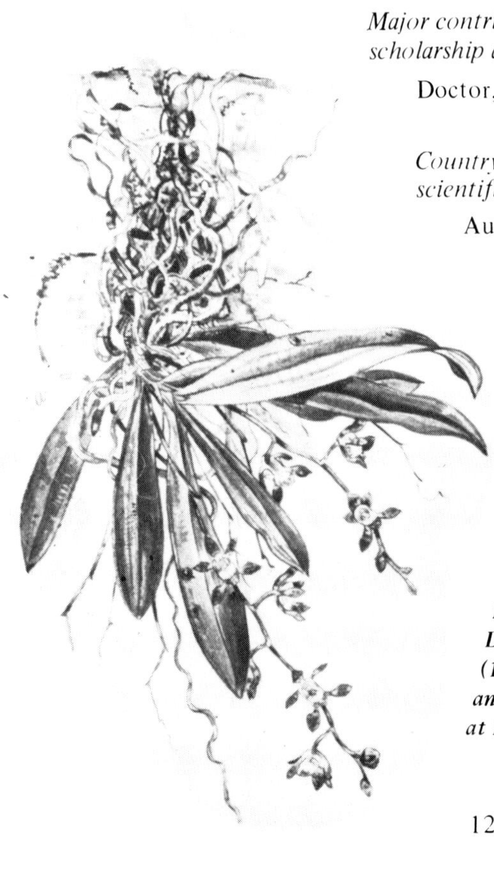

***Sarcochilus bancroftii*, an epiphytic orchid from Mt French, Queensland. Named in honour of Dr THOMAS LANE BANCROFT (1860–1933) medical practitioner and natural historian who worked at Brisbane, Innisfail and Eidsvold.**

BASEDOW, Dr Herbert (1881–1933)

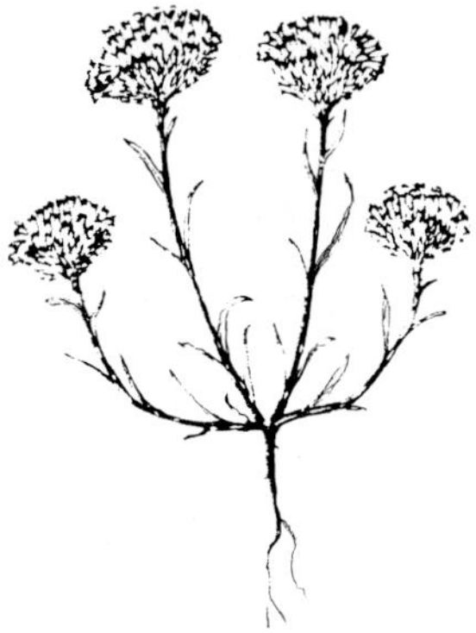

Helichrysum basedowii

Major contributions to medicine, exploration, scholarship and civic life –

Physician, Anthropologist,
Explorer, Geologist,
Parliamentarian,
Natural Historian

Countries of residence and civic and scientific contribution –

Australia (South Australia,
Northern Territory),
Germany

Scientific Name – *Basedowia* spp.

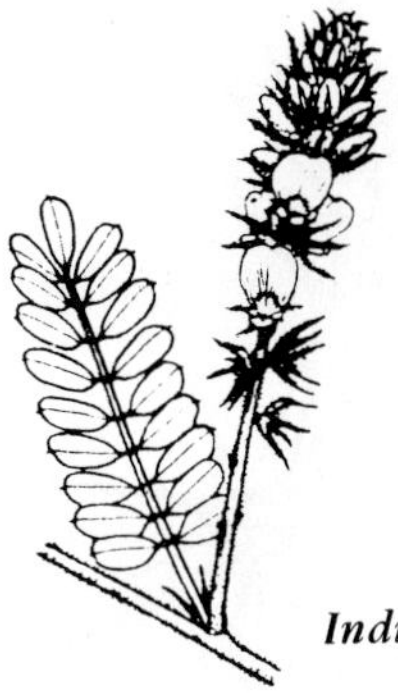

Indigofera basedowii

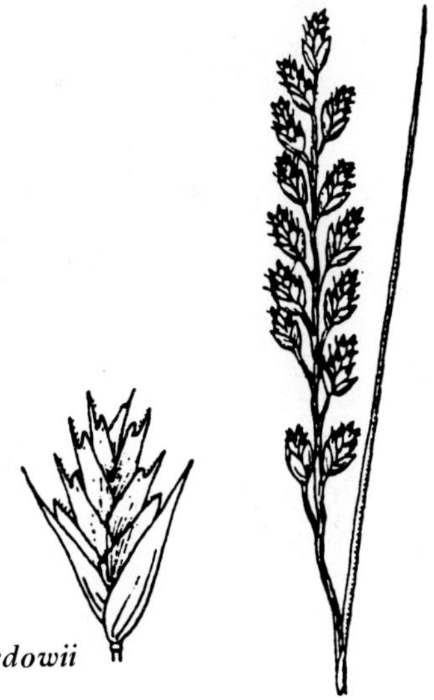

Triodia basedowii

BASSI, Dr Ferdinando (1710–1774)

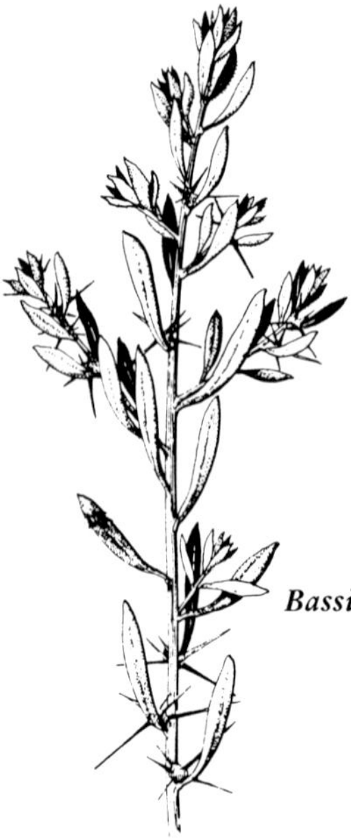

Major contributions to medicine, exploration, scholarship and civic life –

Botanist, Doctor

Country of residence and civic and scientific contribution –

Italy (Bologna)

Scientific Names –

Bassia spp.
Beauveria bassiana (a fungus)

Bassia (syn. ***Sclerolaena***) sp.

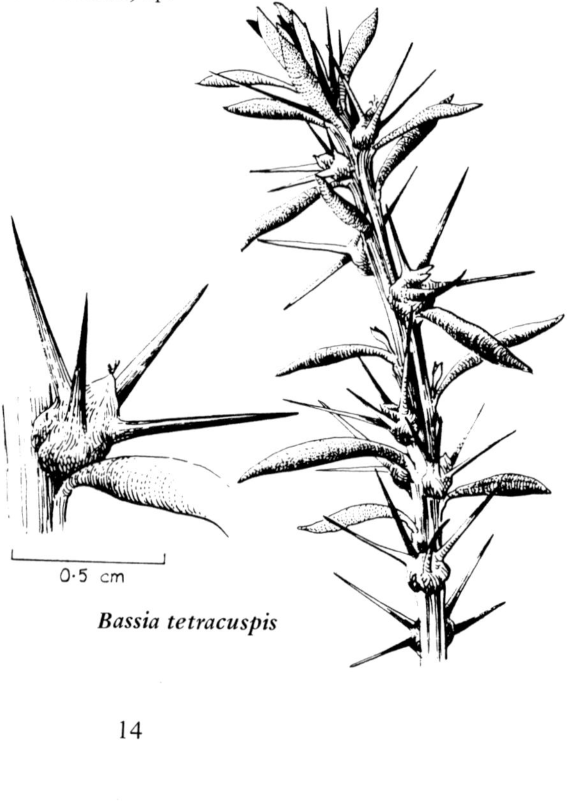

Bassia tetracuspis

BAUHIN, Dr Johann [Jean] (1541–1612)

Major contributions to medicine, exploration, scholarship and civic life –
Botanist, Physician

Countries of residence and civic and scientific contribution –
Switzerland (Basel), France (Montbeliard), Italy

Scientific Name – Bauhinia spp.

BAUHIN, Professor Johann [Jean] Kaspar [Gaspard] (1560–1624) [brother of Johann]

Major contributions to medicine, exploration, scholarship and civic life –
Botanist, Physician, Greek Scholar, Anatomist
Professor of Botany and Anatomy

Countries of residence and civic and scientific contribution –
Switzerland (Basel), Italy (Padua)

Scientific Name – Bauhinia spp.

BAUME, Professor E.F. Antoine (1728–1804)

Major contributions to medicine, exploration, scholarship and civic life –
Apothecary, Chemist, Inventor

Country of residence and civic and scientific contribution –
France (Senlis, Paris)

Scientific Name – Baumea spp.

BECKLER, Dr Hermann (1828–1914)

Major contributions to medicine, exploration, scholarship and civic life –

Physician, Surgeon, Botanist, Explorer

Countries of residence and civic and scientific contribution –

Germany (Munich, Berlin), Australia (Ipswich, Warwick, Tenterfield, Melbourne, Murray-Darling Region)

Scientific Names –

Acacia beckleri
Dendrobium beckleri

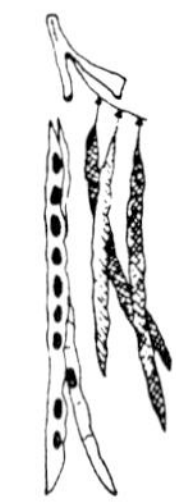

Acacia sp.

BEHR, Professor Hans Hermann (1818–1904)

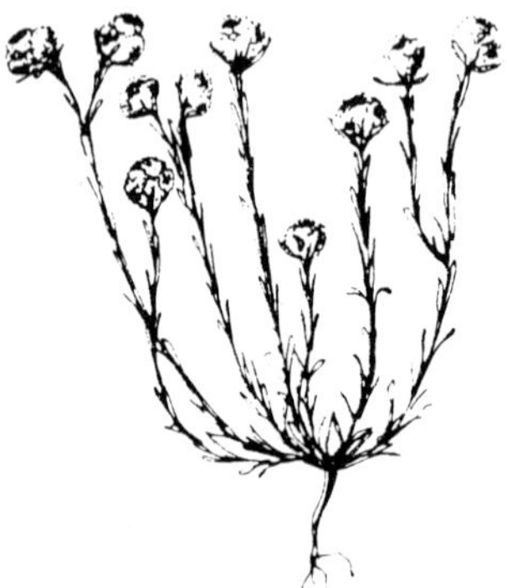

Eriochlamys behrii

Major contributions to medicine, exploration, scholarship and civic life –

Physician, Botanist, Entomologist, Lepidopterist, Poet, Writer, Humorist, Linguist

Countries of residence and civic and scientific contribution –

Germany (Anhalt, Berlin), East Indies (Java, Straits Settlements), Australia (S.Aust. especially Barossa, Gawler, Mt Lofty & Murray River region), Philippines, U.S.A. (California), South Africa

Scientific Names –

Eucalyptus behriana
Senecio behrianus

BEILSCHMIED, Dr Karl Traugott (1793–1848)

Major contributions to medicine, exploration, scholarship and civic life –
Apothecary, Botanist, Linguist

Country of residence and civic and scientific contribution –
Germany (Berlin, Bonn, Schmiedeberg in Schlesien, Ohlau)

Scientific Name – *Beilschmiedia* spp.

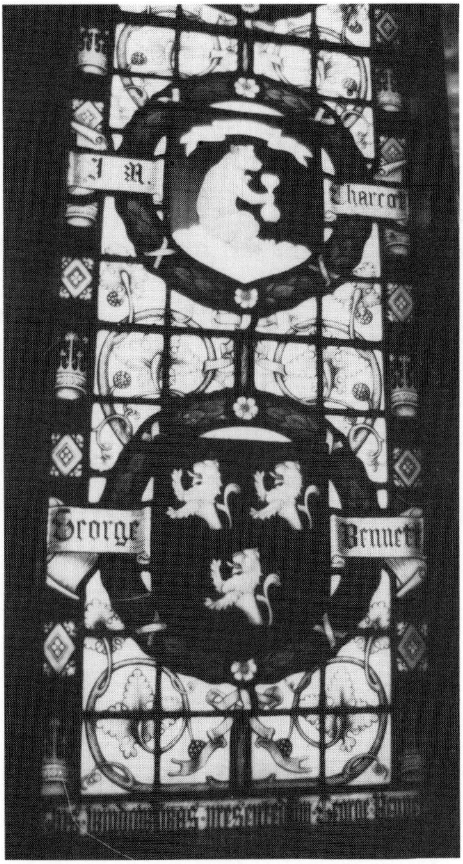

THE BENNETT WINDOW,
in the east stairwell of
The Anderson Stuart Building
(old Faculty of Medicine Building),
University of Sydney.

This stained glass window commemorates Dr GEORGE BENNETT (1804–1893), eminent surgeon, botanist and zoologist of Sydney, and a Founder of the Faculty of Medicine at the University of Sydney.

Photo by the Author, in 1987, by kind permission of Professor Richard Gye, sometime Dean of the Faculty.

BENNETT, Surgeon George (1804–1893)

Major contributions to medicine, exploration, scholarship and civic life –

Surgeon, Botanist, Voyager, Anthropologist, Zoologist, Clinical Teacher, Medical Educator, Writer

Countries of residence and civic and scientific contribution –

England (Plymouth, London), Scotland, Ceylon (Sri Lanka), China, Mauritius, Indonesia, Australia (Queensland, Sydney, Tasmania, South Australia, Norfolk Island), New Zealand

Scientific Names –

Eupomatia bennettii
Flindersia bennettiana

BENNETT, Dr John Joseph (1801–1876)

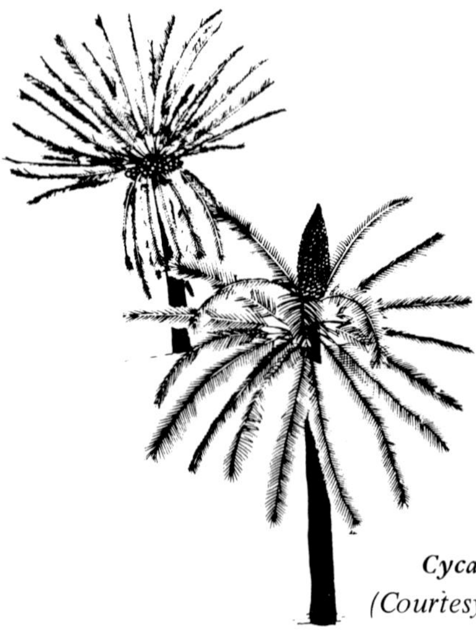

Cycas sp.
(Courtesy of Adi Dunlop, Darwin)

Major contributions to medicine, exploration, scholarship and civic life –

Surgeon, Botanist

Country of residence and civic and scientific contribution –

England (London)

Scientific Name –

Bennettites spp.
(syn. *Cycadeoidea*)

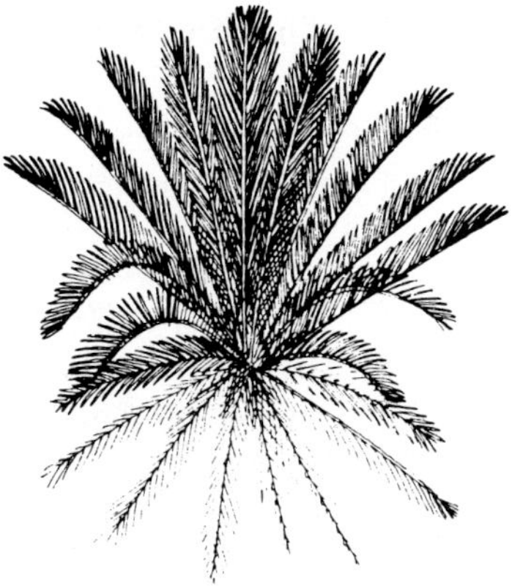

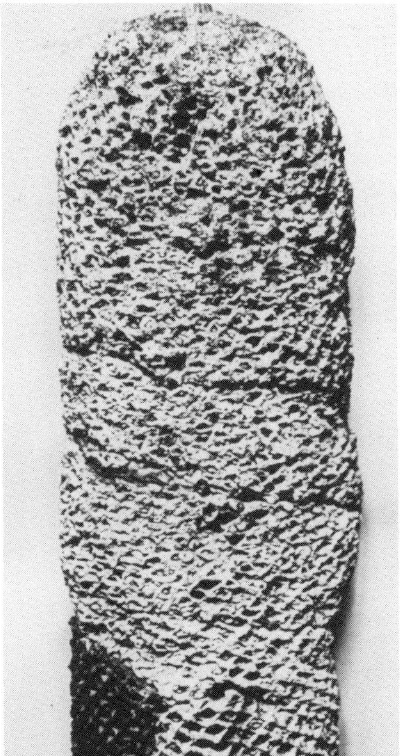

The fossil plant
Cycadeoidea (syn. Bennettites)
gigantea, from Upper Juraassic beds.

The generic synonym commemorates
Dr JOHN JOSEPH BENNETT
(1801–1876) the London
doctor and botanist
who worked on the Australian plant
collections at Kew in the period
1857–1870.

Photo courtesy of Dr Chris Hill,
Department of Palaeontology,
The British Museum of
Natural History.

BERGIUS, Professor Peter Jonas (1730–1790)

Major contributions to medicine, exploration, scholarship and civic life –
Physician, Pharmacist, Naturalist, Botanist

Countries of residence and civic and scientific contribution –
Sweden (Stockholm), South Africa

Scientific Name – *Bergia* spp.

BERRY, Dr Andrew (*fl.* 1784–1819)

Major contributions to medicine, exploration, scholarship and civic life –
Physician, Botanist

Countries of residence and civic and scientific contribution –
Scotland, India (Madras)

Scientific Name – *Berrya* spp.

BERRY, Professor Richard James Arthur (1867–1962)

Major contributions to medicine, exploration, scholarship and civic life –

Anatomist, Anthropologist, Psychiatrist, Dean of Medicine

Countries of residence and civic and scientific contribution –

England (Lancashire), Scotland (Edinburgh, Aberdeen),
Australia (Melbourne)

Scientific Name – *Grevillea berryanus*

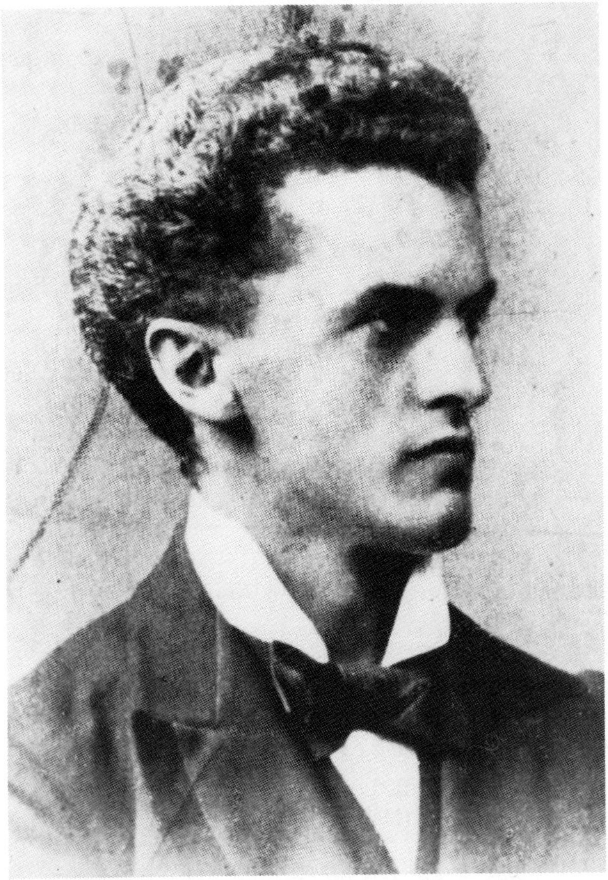

Professor RICHARD JAMES ARTHUR BERRY F.R.S.
(1867–1962),
anatomist, and Dean of Medicine at
Melbourne University.

Photo by W. Crooke of Edinburgh, c. 1900.

de LA BILLARDIERE, Dr Jacques-Julian (Houttou)(1755–1834)

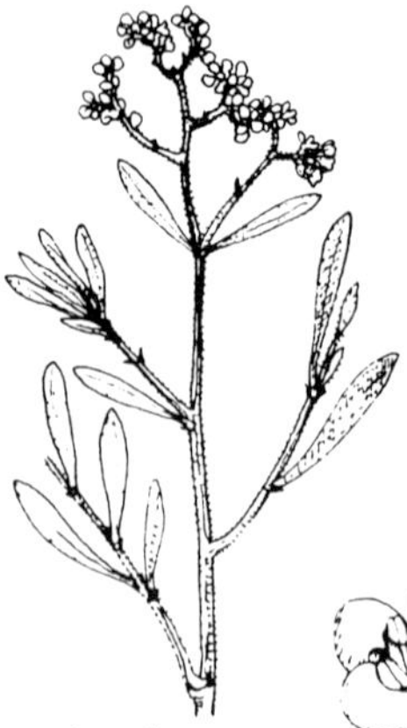

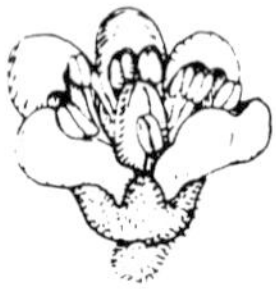

Nitraria billardieri

Major contributions to medicine, exploration, scholarship and civic life –

Doctor, Botanist, Explorer,
Anthropologist

Countries of residence and civic and scientific contribution –

France (Montpellier, Paris),
England, Syria,
Australia (Tasmania, Western Australia)
East Indies, New Caledonia

Scientific Names –

Billardiera spp.
Nitraria billardieri

BIRD, Dr Samuel Dougan (1832–1904)

Major contributions to medicine, exploration, scholarship and civic life –

Physician, Military Surgeon, University Lecturer

Countries of residence and civic and scientific contribution –

England (Lowestoft, London), Russia
Turkey, Australia (Melbourne)

Scientific Name – Calytrix birdii

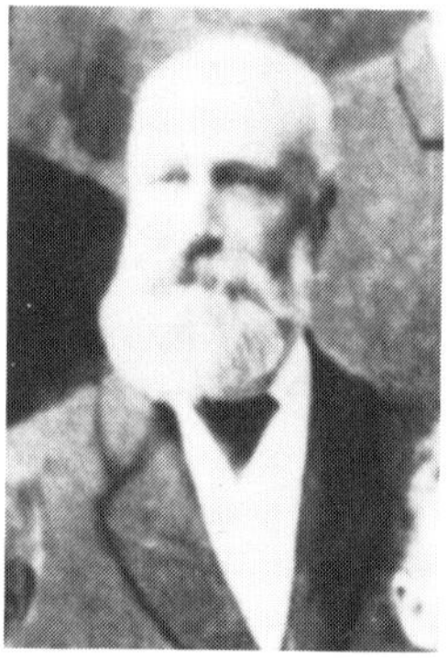

Dr SAMUEL DOUGAN BIRD (1832–1904), Physician, Military Surgeon, and University teacher, of Melbourne. The plant Calytrix birdii, known as Bird's Fringe-myrtle, commemorates him.

BLACK, Dr Thomas (*c.* 1803–1894)

Major contributions to medicine, exploration, scholarship and civic life –
Physician, Botanist

Country of residence and civic and scientific contribution –
Australia (Melbourne)

Scientific Name – Anthotroche blackii

BLACKALL, Dr William (1876–1941)

Major contributions to medicine, exploration, scholarship and civic life –
Physician, Psychiatrist, Surgeon, Botanist,
Military Surgeon, Obstetrician, Paediatrician

Countries of residence and civic and scientific contribution –
England (Oxford, London),
Australia (Perth)

Scientific Name –
Blackallia spp.
(also the genus *Nigromnia* – a Latinized form of the above)

de BLAINVILLE, Professor Henri Marie Ducrotay (1778–1850)

Major contributions to medicine, exploration, scholarship and civic life –
Doctor, Natural Historian, Ichthyologist, Paleobotanist

Country of residence and civic and scientific contribution –
France (Paris)

Scientific Name – Blainvillea spp.

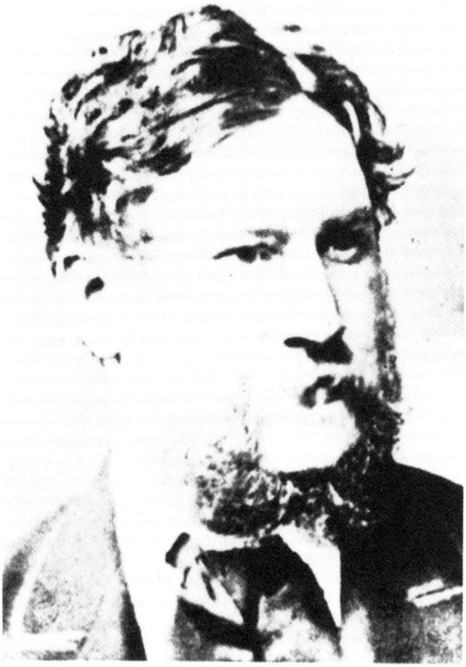

Dr JOHN BLAIR (1834–1887) surgeon, obstetrician, writer and art collector, of Melbourne.

His memorial is the Australian plant Rhodamnia blairiana.

Photo, courtesy of Dr Ann Mitchell, and the Alfred Hospital, Melbourne, of which he was the founder.

BLAIR, Dr John (1834–1887)

Major contributions to medicine, exploration, scholarship and civic life –

Surgeon, Obstetrician, Medical Patron, Writer, Art Collector

Countries of residence and civic and scientific contribution –

Scotland (Glasgow, Edinburgh)
Australia (Melbourne)

Scientific Name – Rhodamnia blairiana

BLEASDALE, Rev. Dr John Ignatius (1822–1884)

Major contributions to medicine, exploration, scholarship and civic life –

Catholic Priest, Military Chaplain, Microscopist,
Patron of Medicine and Health,
Botanist, viticulturalist

Countries of residence and civic and scientific contribution –

England (Birmingham),
Australia (Geelong, Melbourne),
United States (California)

Scientific Name – *Bleasdalea* spp.

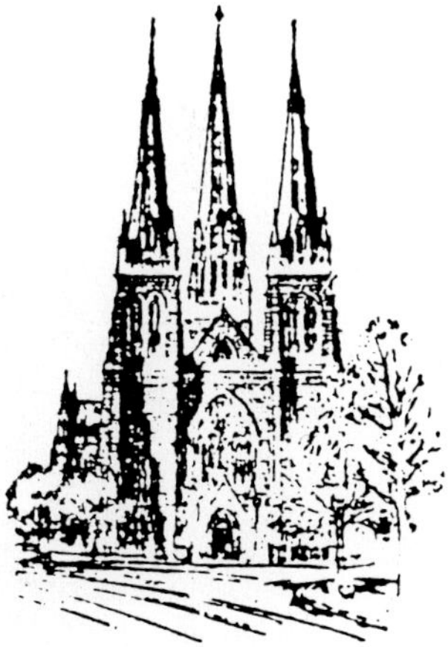

BLUME, Dr Carl Ludwig (1796–1862)

Major contributions to medicine, exploration, scholarship and civic life –

Physician, Botanist, Illustrator

Countries of residence and civic and scientific contribution –

Germany (Brunswick),
Holland (Leiden),
Indonesia (esp. Java)

Scientific Name – *Blumea* spp.

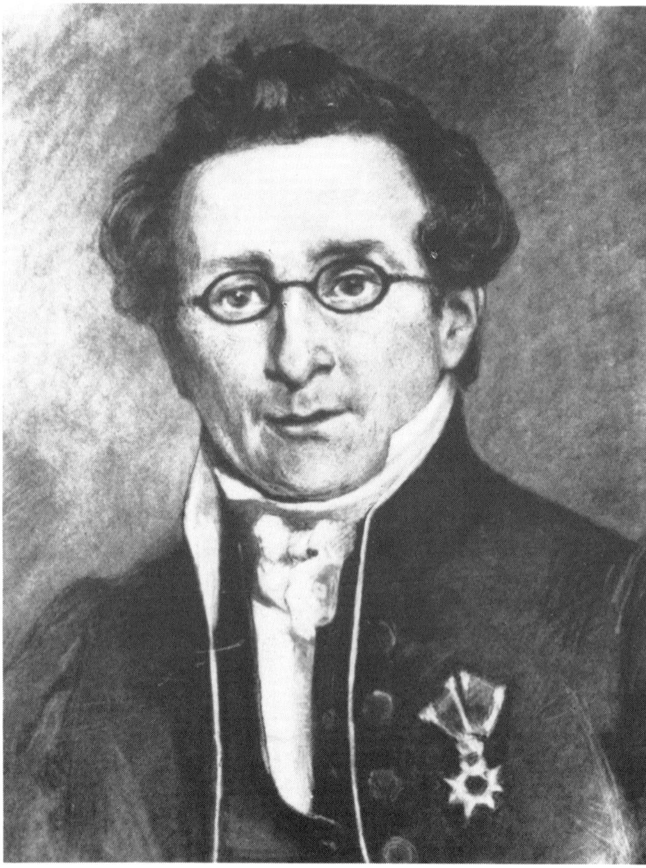

Dr CARL LUDWIG BLUME
(1796–1862),
physician and botanist, whose name is commemorated in the genus Blumea, of which some twelve species are native to Australia.

Photo, courtesy of the Hunt Institute for Botanical Documentation, Carnegie Mellon University, Pittsburgh, and Ms Anita Karg.

BOEHMER, Professor Georg Rudolph (1723–1803)

Major contributions to medicine, exploration, scholarship and civic life –

Physician, Anatomist, Botanist

Countries of residence and civic and scientific contribution –

Germany (Wittenburg)

Scientific Name – Boehmeria spp.

BOERHAAVE, Professor Hermann (1668–1738)

Major contributions to medicine, exploration, scholarship and civic life –

Physician, Botanist, Chemist, Teacher and Medical Educator

Countries of residence and civic and scientific contribution –

Holland (Leiden)

Scientific Name – Boerhavia spp.

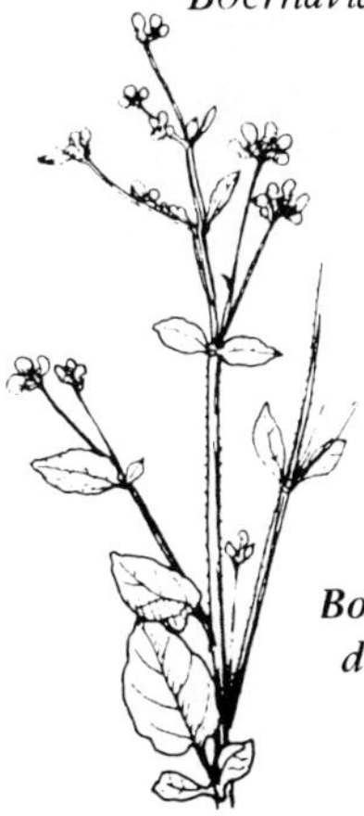

Boerhavia diffusa

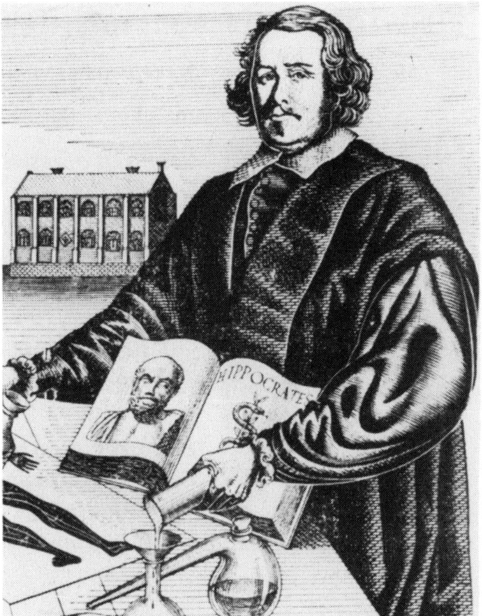

Professor Hermann Boerhaave (1668-1738) of Leiden, Holland. One of the greatest teachers in the history of medicine. An eminent botanist also, his name is commemorated in several Australian species of Boerhavia. Photo courtesy of 'A Student Anthology'.

BONAMY, Dr Francois (1710–1786)(also BONAMI)

Major contributions to medicine, exploration, scholarship and civic life –

Doctor, Botanist, University Rector, Patron of Science

Countries of residence and civic and scientific contribution –

France (Montpellier, Nantes)

Scientific Name – Bonamia spp.

BOSISTO, ("Dr") Joseph (1827–1898)

Major contributions to medicine, exploration, scholarship and civic life –

Pharmacist, Chemist, Politician

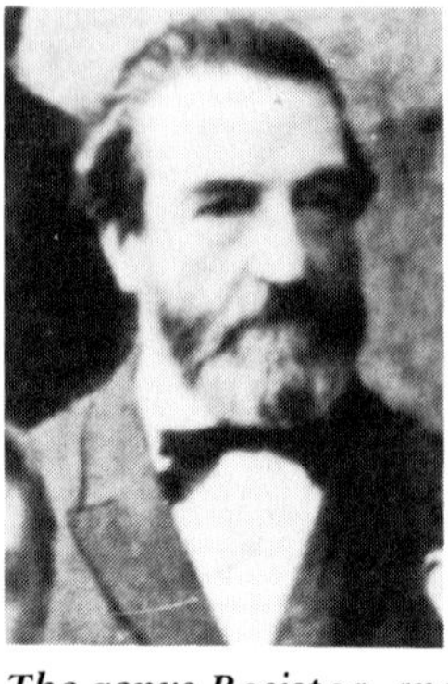

Countries of residence and civic and scientific contribution –

England (Berkshire),
Australia (Adelaide, Melbourne)

Scientific Names –

Bosistoa spp.
Eucalyptus bosistoana

Dr Joseph Bosisto (1827–1898) Pharmacist, chemist and politician of Melbourne. The genus Bosistoa, and a beautiful species of Australian gumtree, Eucalyptus bosistoana form his timeless memorials.

de BOSSIEU de la Martini re, Dr Joseph (1754–1788)

Major contributions to medicine, exploration, scholarship and civic life –

Naval Surgeon, Botanist

Countries of residence and civic and scientific contribution –

France, Australia (Botany Bay), South Pacific (perished in Melanesia)

Scientific Name – Bossiaea spp.

BOUCHARDAT, Professor Apollinaire (1806–1886)

Major contributions to medicine, exploration, scholarship and civic life –

Doctor, Botanist, Pharmacologist, Professor of Medicine

Countries of residence and civic and scientific contribution –

France (Paris)

Scientific Name – Bouchardatia neurococca (a monotypic genus)

BOURJOT, Dr A. (? – ?)

Major contributions to medicine, exploration, scholarship and civic life –

Doctor, Botanist (esp. Eucalypts)

Countries of residence and civic and scientific contribution –

Algeria

Scientific Name – Flindersia bourjotiana

BREYNE, Dr Johann Philipp (1680–1764)

Major contributions to medicine, exploration, scholarship and civic life –

Doctor, Botanist

Countries of residence and civic and scientific contribution –

Poland (Gdansk), Ceylon (Sri Lanka), Spain, Italy (Ancona)

Scientific Name – Breynia spp.

BROWN, Surgeon Robert (1773–1858)

Major contributions to medicine, exploration, scholarship and civic life –

Surgeon, Military Surgeon,
Botanist ("Father of Australian Botany")
Explorer, Microscopist, Librarian

Countries of residence and civic and scientific contribution –

Scotland (Montrose, Aberdeen, Edinburgh)
Ireland, Australia (W.A.; N.S.W.; circumnavigated Australia with Matthew Flinders 1802-3; Tasmania), England (London)

Scientific Names –

Brunonia australis (a monotypic genus)
Brunoniella spp.
Rumex brownii

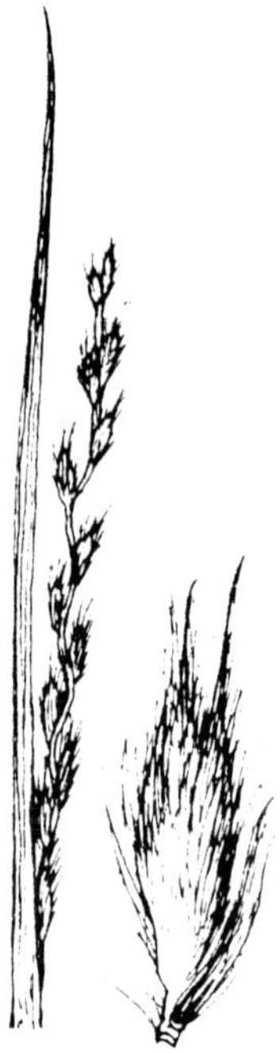

Digitaria brownii

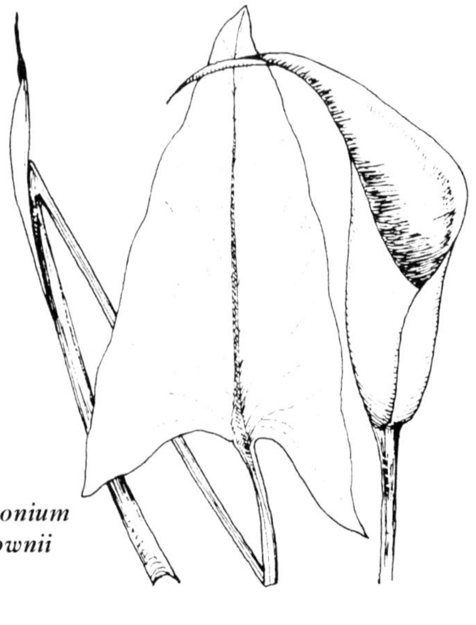

Typhonium brownii

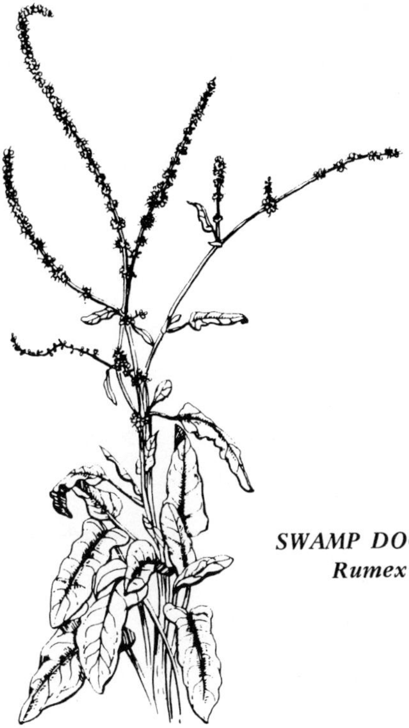

SWAMP DOCK – Rumex brownii

BUCHANAN–HAMILTON, (né BUCHANAN) Surgeon Francis (1762–1829)

Major contributions to medicine, exploration, scholarship and civic life –

Surgeon, Physician, Explorer, Botanist

Countries of residence and civic and scientific contribution –

Scotland (Perthshire), India (Calcutta, Bengal, Andaman Islands, Mysore), Nepal, Burma (now Myanmarh)

Scientific Name – Buchanania spp.

BURCKHARD, Dr Joseph Heinrich (1676–1738)

Major contributions to medicine, exploration, scholarship and civic life –
Physician, Botanist

Countries of residence and civic and scientific contribution –
Germany (Wolfenbuttel)

Scientific Name – *Burchardia* spp.

BURSER, Professor Joachim (1583–1639)

Major contributions to medicine, exploration, scholarship and civic life –
Doctor, Botanist, Professor of Medicine

Countries of residence and civic and scientific contribution –
Denmark (Sors)

Scientific Name – *Bursera* spp. (syn. *Canarium*)

BYNOE, Surgeon Benjamin (1803–1865)

Major contributions to medicine, exploration, scholarship and civic life –
Naval Surgeon, Natural Historian, Plant Collector, Explorer and Voyager

Countries of residence and civic and scientific contribution –
England, Australia (Western Australia, Bass Strait, New South Wales)

Scientific Name – *Acacia bynoeana*

CAESALPINO, Professor Andrea (1519–1603)

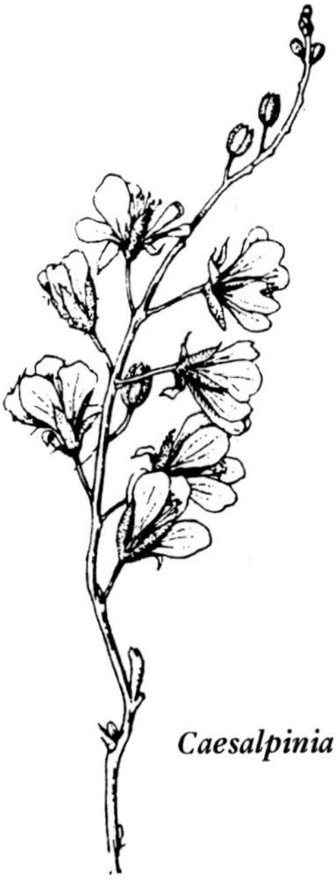

Major contributions to medicine, exploration, scholarship, and civic life –

Physician, Botanist, Gardener, Professor of Medicine,

Countries of residence and civic and scientific contribution –

Italy (Pisa, Roma)

Scientific Name –

Caesalpinia spp.

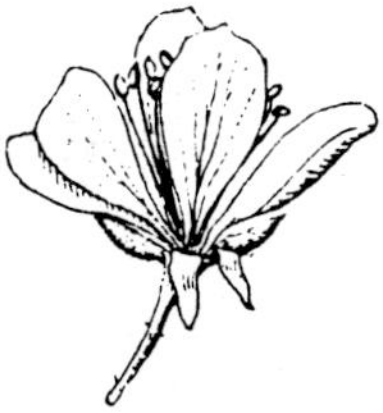

Caesalpinia sp.

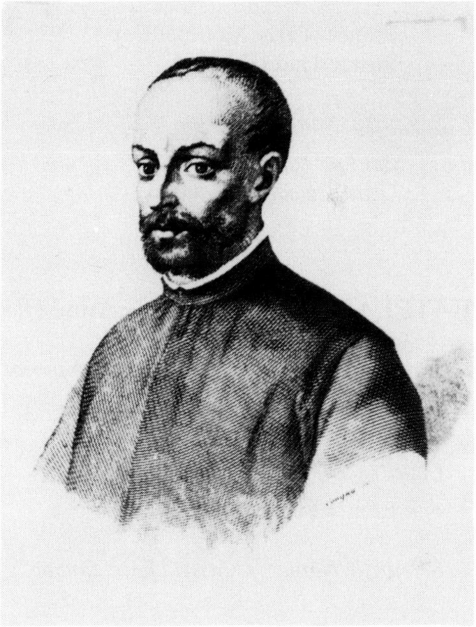

Professore Andrea Caesalpino (1519–1603).
Physician and botanist, and Professor of Medicine at Pisa.

The family CAESALPINIACEAE contains genera of Bauhinia, Cassia and Caesalpinia native to Australia.

Engraving courtesy of the Museo Botanico, Florence.

CADET de GASSICOURT, Dr Charles-Louis (1769–1821)

Major contributions to medicine, exploration, scholarship and civic life –

Apothecary, Lexicographer

Countries of residence and civic and scientific contribution –

France (Paris)

Scientific Name – *Cadetia* spp.

de CANDOLLE, Professor Augustin Pyramus (1778–1841)

Major contributions to medicine, exploration, scholarship and civic life –

Doctor, Botanist, Herbarium Curator,
Writer, Taxonomist

Countries of residence and civic and scientific contribution –

France (Paris, Montpellier)
Switzerland (Geneva)

Scientific Names –

Banksia candolleana
Grevillea candolleana

CHATELAIN, Marie Francois Anne (*fl. c.* 1825)

Major contributions to medicine, exploration, scholarship and civic life –

Pharmacist, Naval Apothecary

Countries of residence and civic and scientific contribution –

France (Toulon)

Scientific Name – *Cassia chatelainiana*

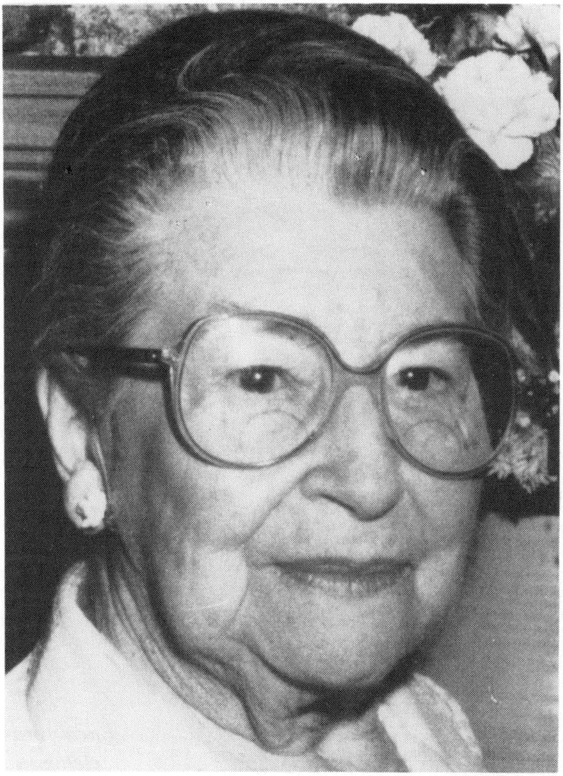

LADY CILENTO (Dr PHYLLIS CILENTO)
(1894–1987).
One of Australia's most famous doctors of modern times – an advocate of equal opportunities for women, and vigorous writer on mothercraft and paediatric issues.

CILENTO, Lady (Dr Phyllis) (1894–1987)

Major contributions to medicine, exploration, scholarship and civic life –

Doctor, Paediatrician, Writer, Champion of Women's Rights

Countries of residence and civic and scientific contribution –

Australia (Adelaide, Brisbane), England (London),
United States of America (New York)

Scientific Name – Hibiscus rosa-sinensis "Lady Cilento"

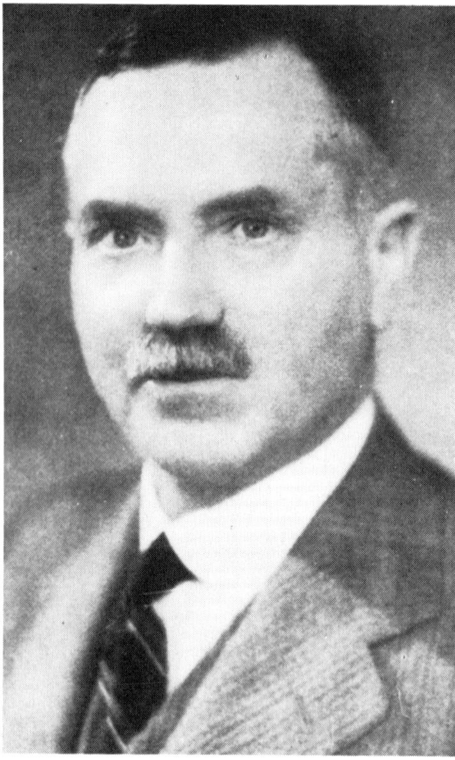

Professor (later, after 1964, Sir) JOHN BURTON CLELAND (1878–1971).

Eminent pathologist and natural historian, of Adelaide. His name is recorded in many species of Australian plants, including one common spinifex of central Australia, Triodia clelandii.

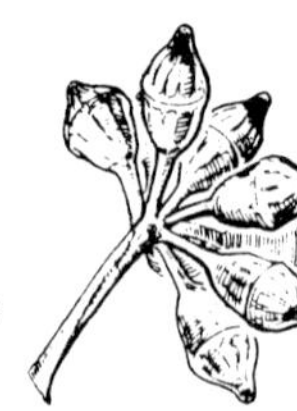

Eucalyptus clelandii

CLELAND, Professor Sir John Burton (1878–1971)

Major contributions to medicine, exploration, scholarship and civic life –

Pathologist, Physician, Natural Historian, Anthropologist, University Teacher

Countries of residence and civic and scientific contribution –

Australia (Adelaide, Sydney), England (London), Scotland (Glasgow)

Scientific Names –

Eucalyptus clelandii
Triodia clelandii

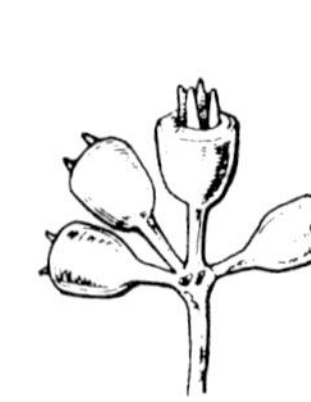

COATES, Surgeon John (1812–1863)

Major contributions to medicine, exploration, scholarship and civic life –

Surgeon, Microscopist, Politician

Countries of residence and civic and scientific contribution –

Australia (Melbourne)

Scientific Name – Hibiscus coatesii

COLDEN, Dr Cadwallader (1688–1776)

Major contributions to medicine, exploration, scholarship and civic life –

Physician, Botanist, Mathematician, Meteorologist, Surveyor, Lieutenant-Governor (of New York), Historian and Writer

Countries of residence and civic and scientific contribution –

Scotland (Edinburgh), England (London), Ireland, United States of America (Pennsylvania, New York)

Scientific Name – Coldenia procumbens (Sole species in Australia)

COMMELIN, Professor Caspar (1667–1731)

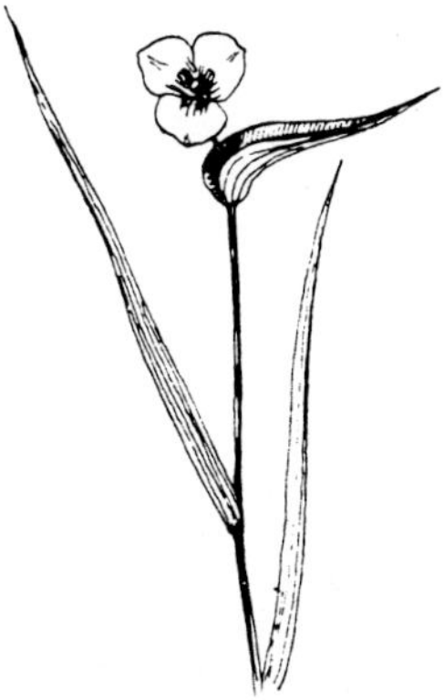

Commelina cyanea

Major contributions to medicine, exploration, scholarship and civic life –

Physician, Botanist, Teacher, Writer

Countries of residence and civic and scientific contribution –

Holland (Leiden, Amsterdam)

Scientific Name –

Commelina spp.

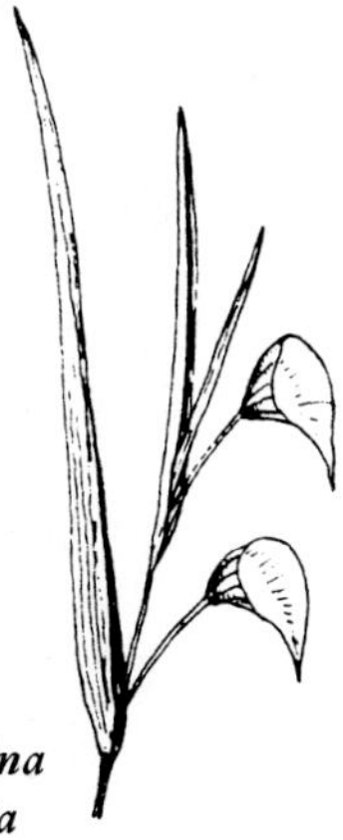

Commelina ensifolia

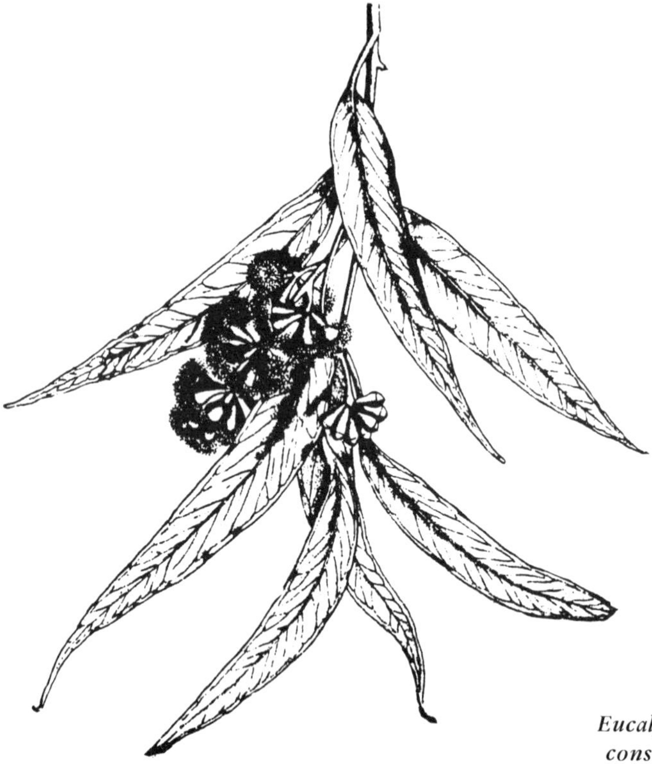

Eucalyptus consideniana

CONSIDEN, Surgeon Denis (*c.* **1775–1815**)

Major contributions to medicine, exploration, scholarship and civic life –

Naval Surgeon, Army Surgeon, Doctor, Natural Historian

Countries of residence and civic and scientific contribution –

Ireland (County Clare), Scotland (Edinburgh),
Australia (Sydney – First Fleet Surgeon), South Africa

Scientific Name – Eucalyptus consideniana

CORDUS, Dr Eurich (1484–1535)

Major contributions to medicine, exploration, scholarship and civic life –
Physician, Poet, Philosopher, Teacher, Botanist

Countries of residence and civic and scientific contribution –
Germany (Erfurt, Marburg, Bremen)

Scientific Name – *Cordia* spp.

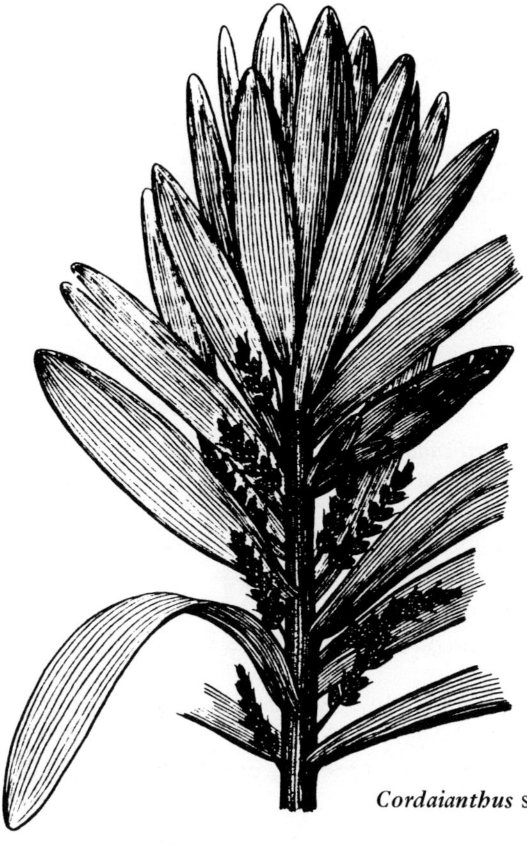

Cordaianthus sp.

CROWE, Surgeon James (1750–1807)

Major contributions to medicine, exploration, scholarship and civic life –

Surgeon, Botanist

Countries of residence and civic and scientific contribution –

England (Norfolk)

Scientific Name – *Crowea* spp.

CURDIE, Dr Daniel (1810–1884)

Major contributions to medicine, exploration, scholarship and civic life –

Doctor, Explorer, Pastoralist, Botanist,
Teacher, University Senator, Town Councillor

Countries of residence and civic and scientific contribution –

Scotland (Arran),
Australia (Geelong District)

Scientific Names –

Curdiea spp.
Hymenena curdieana
Limosella curdieana

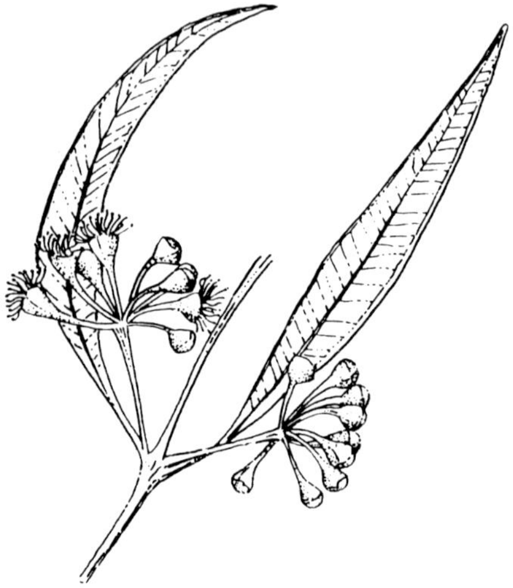

DAINTRY, Edwin (1814–1887)

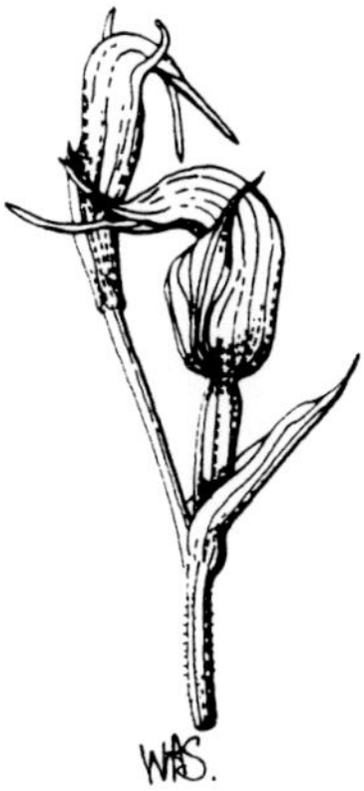

Major contributions to medicine, exploration, scholarship and civic life –

Medical Student, Solicitor, Librarian, Botanist

Countries of residence and civic and scientific contribution –

England (Sussex)
Australia (Sydney)

Scientific Name –

Pterostylis daintreana

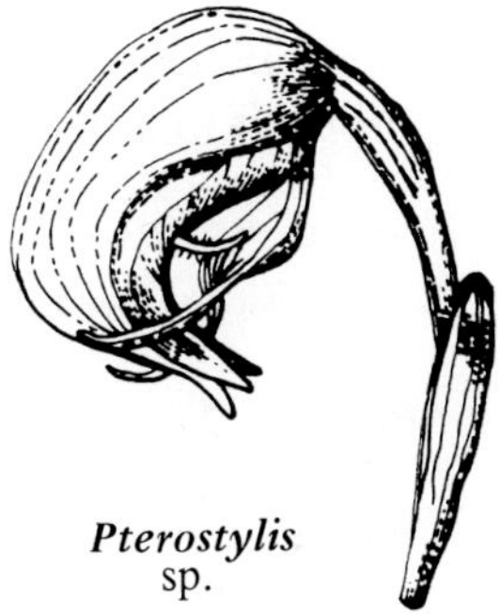

Pterostylis sp.

DALBERG, Dr Nils E. (1736–1820)

Major contributions to medicine, exploration, scholarship and civic life –

Physician

Countries of residence and civic and scientific contribution –

Sweden (Stockholm)

Scientific Name –

Dalbergia densa (only species in Australia)

DARWIN, Charles (1809–1882)

Major contributions to medicine, exploration, scholarship and civic life –

Medical Student, Natural Historian, Explorer, Scientist, Writer

Countries of residence and civic and scientific contribution –

England (Downe, in Kent), South America, Pacific, Australia (Sydney, Hobart)

Scientific Name –

Cyttaria darwinii (a fungus)

DARWIN, Dr Erasmus (1731–1802) (Grandfather of Charles Darwin)

Major contributions to medicine, exploration, scholarship and civic life –

Physician, Botanist, Poet, Gardener

Countries of residence and civic and scientific contribution –

England (Lichfield, Derby)

Scientific Names –

Darwinia spp.
Homorathus darwinioides

DAVIES, Dr Charles (1814–1888)

Major contributions to medicine, exploration, scholarship and civic life –

Doctor, Pastoralist, Politician, Natural Historian

Countries of residence and civic and scientific contribution –

Wales, France, Australia (Adelaide)

Scientific Name – Velleia daviesii

DEERING, Dr George Charles (*c.* 1695–1749)

Major contributions to medicine, exploration, scholarship and civic life –

Doctor, Historian, Botanist, Army Surgeon

Countries of residence and civic and scientific contribution –

Germany (Hamburg, Saxony), Holland (Leiden),
England (London, Nottingham)

Scientific Name – *Deeringia* spp.

DENMARK, Surgeon Alexander (*fl.* 1797–1830)

Major contributions to medicine, exploration, scholarship and civic life –

Naval Surgeon

Countries of residence and civic and scientific contribution –

England (Gosport)

Scientific Name – *Meeboldina denmarkica*

DEPLANCHE, Surgeon Emile (1824–1875)

Major contributions to medicine, exploration, scholarship and civic life –

Naval Surgeon, Botanist, Zoologist, Anthropologist

Countries of residence and civic and scientific contribution –

France (Caen, Normandy), Crimea, West Indies (Cayenne)
South Pacific, New Caledonia

Scientific Name – *Deplanchea* spp.

DESCHAMPS, Surgeon Louis Auguste (1765–1842)

Major contributions to medicine, exploration, scholarship and civic life –

Naval Surgeon, Naturalist, Explorer

Countries of residence and civic and scientific contribution –

France, Indonesia (Java), Australia (Tasmania, Western Australia)

Scientific Name –

Deschampsia caespitosa
(one Australian species in this group)

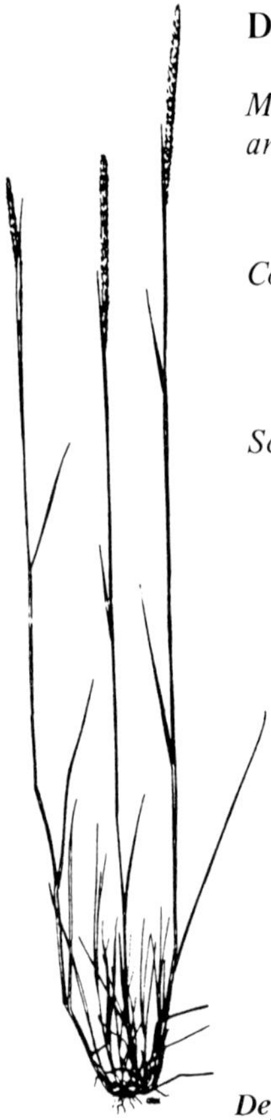

DEYEUX, Professor Nicolas (1753–1837)

Major contributions to medicine, exploration, scholarship and civic life –

Pharmacist, Botanist

Countries of residence and civic and scientific contribution –

France

Scientific Name – Deyeuxia spp.

Deyeuxia imbricata

DICKSON, Dr Robert (1804–1875)

Major contributions to medicine, exploration, scholarship and civic life –

Physician, Paediatrician, Botanist, Teacher, Patron of Arts and Music

Countries of residence and civic and scientific contribution –

England (London, Slough), Scotland (Dumphries, Edinburgh)

Scientific Name – Chorizema dicksonii

DILLENIUS, Professor Johann Jacob (1684–1747)

Major contributions to medicine, exploration, scholarship and civic life –
Physician, Botanist, Professor of Botany

Countries of residence and civic and scientific contribution –
Germany (Giessen), England (Oxford)

Scientific Name – Dillenia alata

DIOSCORIDES, Pedanios (1st Century A.D.)

Major contributions to medicine, exploration, scholarship and civic life –
Physician, Army Physician, Herbalist, Botanist, Pharmacologist

Countries of residence and civic and scientific contribution –
Greece, Cilicia (now part of Turkey in Asia Minor)

Scientific Name – Dioscorea spp.

DODOENS, Professor Rembert (1517–1585)

Major contributions to medicine, exploration, scholarship and civic life –
Physician, Physiologist, Herbalist, Botanist, Medical Teacher

Countries of residence and civic and scientific contribution –
Belgium (Malines), Holland (Leiden), Austria (Vienna), Germany (Cologne)

Scientific Name – Dodonaea spp.

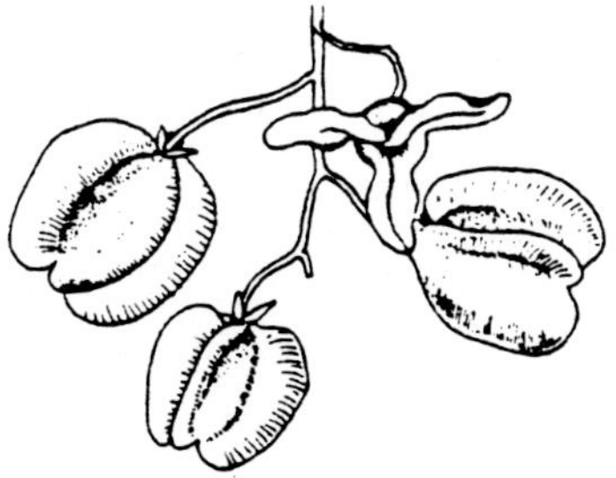

Dodonaea lanceolata

DURRINGTON, Dr Lorraine (now Dr Lorraine Tan) (Born 1948)

Major contributions to medicine, exploration, scholarship and civic life –
Doctor, Botanist

Countries of residence and civic and scientific contribution –
Australia (Brisbane, Buderim)

Scientific Name –
Durringtonia paludosa (a monotypic genus)

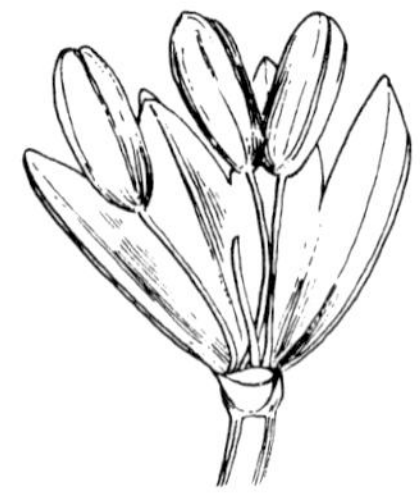

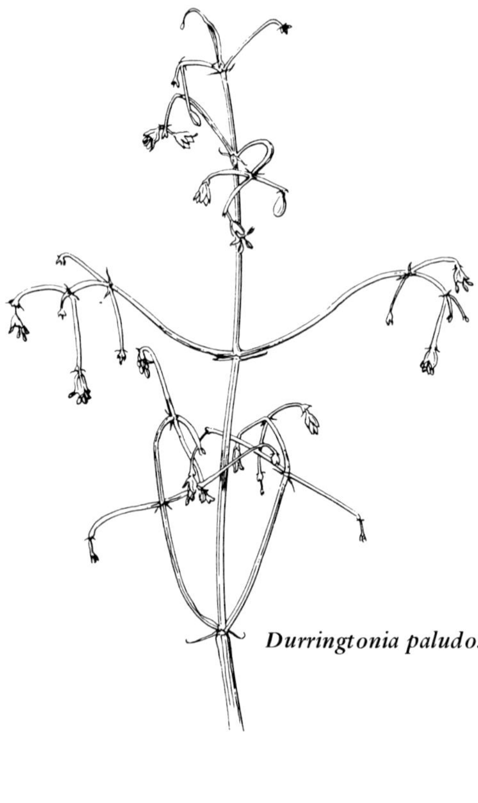

Durringtonia paludosa

EBERMAIER, Dr Johann Erdmann Christian (1767–1825)

Major contributions to medicine, exploration, scholarship and civic life –

Apothecary, Doctor, Herbalist

Countries of residence and civic and scientific contribution –

Austria (Osnabruck), Germany (Dusseldorf)

Scientific Name – Ebermaiera glauca (the only species in Australia)

ELSEY, Surgeon Joseph Ravenscroft (1834–1857)

Major contributions to medicine, exploration, scholarship and civic life –

Surgeon, Explorer, Naturalist, Ornithologist

Countries of residence and civic and scientific contribution –

England (London), Australia (Northern Territory, Queensland), West Indies (St Kitts)

Scientific Name – Ripogonum elseyanum

EMBLING, Dr Thomas (1814–1893)

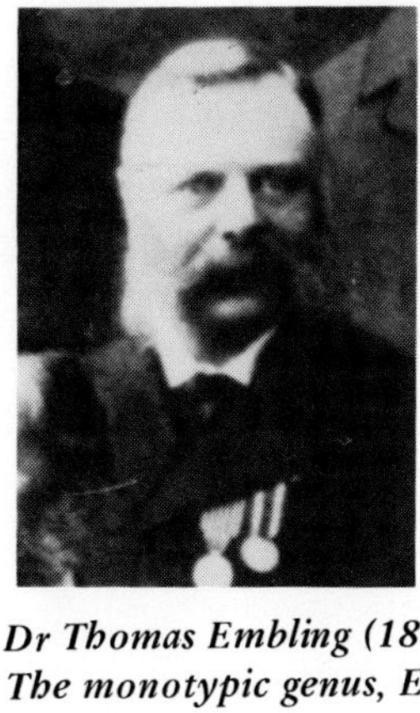

Major contributions to medicine, exploration, scholarship and civic life –

Apothecary, Surgeon, Psychiatrist, Politician

Countries of residence and civic and scientific contribution –

England (London), Australia (Melbourne)

Scientific Name – Emblingia calceoliflora (a monotypic genus)

Dr Thomas Embling (1814–1893), surgeon and politician of Melbourne. The monotypic genus, Emblingia calceoliflora, commemorates his name.

EUPHORBUS, (First Century B.C.)

Major contributions to medicine, exploration, scholarship and civic life –

Countries of residence and civic and scientific contribution –

Greece , Africa (Mauritania)

Scientific Name – Euphorbia spp.

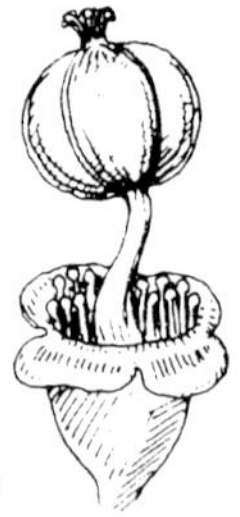

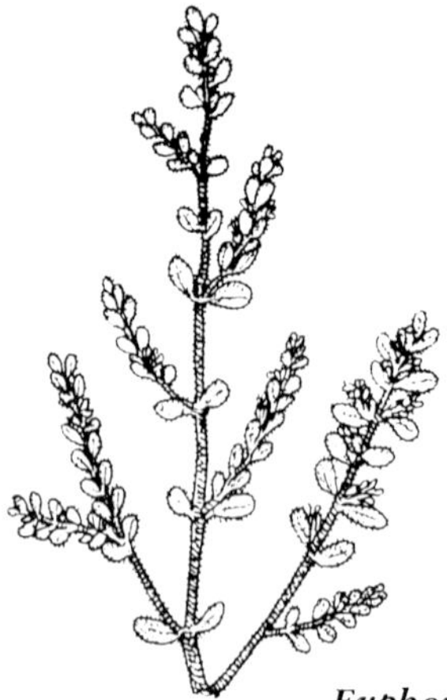

Euphorbia australis

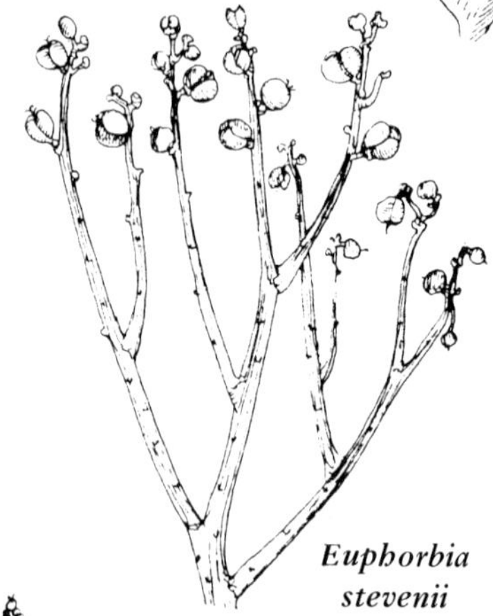

Euphorbia stevenii

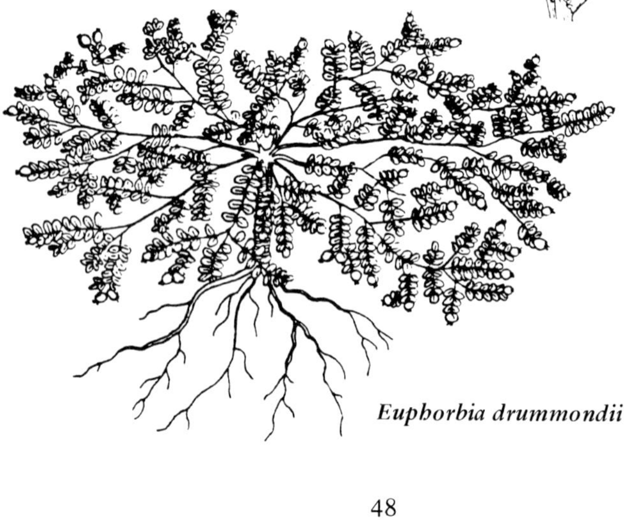

Euphorbia drummondii

FAGRAEUS, Dr Jonas Theodor (1729–1797)

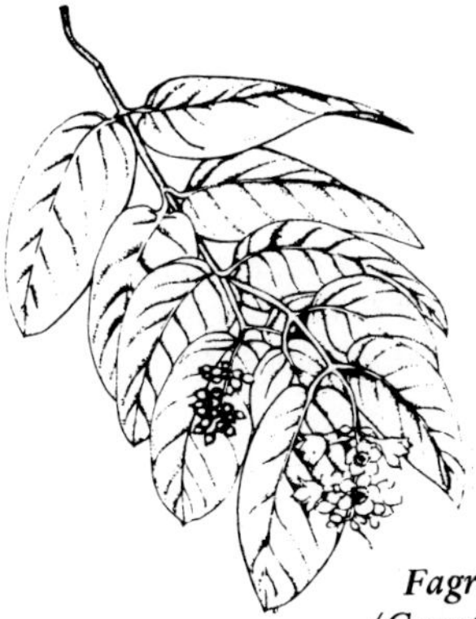

Major contributions to medicine, exploration, scholarship and civic life –

Doctor, Botanist, Natural Historian

Countries of residence and civic and scientific contribution –

Sweden (Uppsala)

Scientific Name – *Fagraea* spp.

Fagraea racemosa
(Courtesy of Adi Dunlop, Darwin)

FARRAGE, Dr William (1821–1876)

Major contributions to medicine, exploration, scholarship and civic life –

Surgeon

Countries of residence and civic and scientific contribution –

Scotland (Glasgow), Australia (Melbourne),
England (Chippenham)

Scientific Name – *Radyera farragei*

FARRER, William James (1845–1906)

Major contributions to medicine, exploration, scholarship and civic life –

Medical Student, Wheat-breeder, Geneticist

Countries of residence and civic and scientific contribution –

England (Westmoreland, London, Cambridge), Australia (Thorwa, near what is now Canberra, Murrumbidgee River Region)

Scientific Name –

Triticum vulgare (Common Wheat)
Farrer's "Federation"

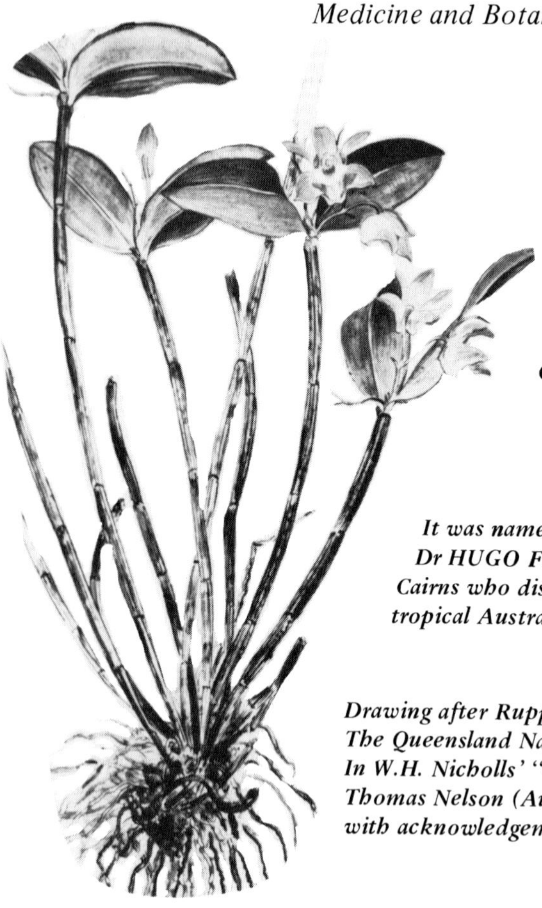

Dendrobium fleckeri Rupp, the epiphytic orchid of Mt Spurgeon, Mt Bartle Frere and Mt Bellenden Ker in the Cairns hinterland, Queensland.

It was named after its discoverer, Dr HUGO FLECKER (1884–1957), of Cairns who discovered many new species of tropical Australian flora.

Drawing after Rupp MMR and White CT, The Queensland Naturalist 1937; 10:25-26. In W.H. Nicholls' "Orchids of Australia", Thomas Nelson (Australia) with acknowledgements.

FLECKER, Dr Hugo (1884–1957)

Major contributions to medicine, exploration, scholarship and civic life –

Doctor, Army Doctor, Radiologist, Radiotherapist,
Botanist, Zoologist

Countries of residence and civic and scientific contribution –

Australia (Sydney, Cairns), Egypt, France

Scientific Names –

Dendrobium fleckeri
Liparis fleckeri

FLEMING, Dr John (1747–1829)

Major contributions to medicine, exploration, scholarship and civic life –

Physician, Botanist, Parliamentarian

Countries of residence and civic and scientific contribution –

England (London), India (Bengal, Punjab, Calcutta), Pakistan

Scientific Name – Flemingia spp.

FORSTER, Professor Johann Georg Adam (1754–1794) (Son of Johann Reinhold)

Major contributions to medicine, exploration, scholarship and civic life –

Doctor, Explorer, Botanist, Natural Historian, Writer, Revolutionary

Countries of residence and civic and scientific contribution –

Germany (Kassel, Mainz), Russia, England (London), Australia, Poland (Vilna)

Scientific Names –

Forstera bellidifolia (only one species in Australia, in Tasmania)

Microseris forsteri

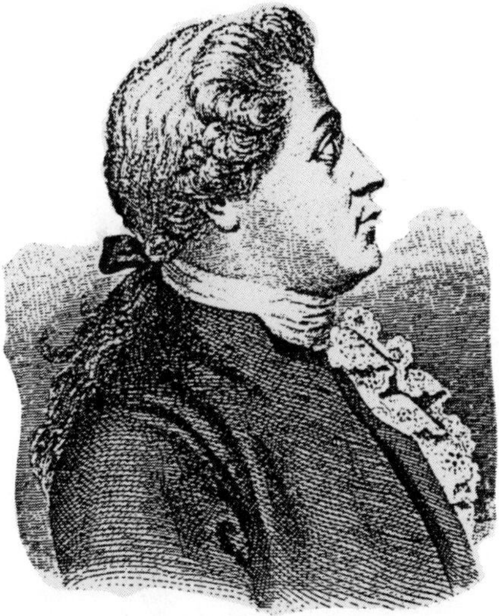

Professor Johann Georg Adam Forster (1754–1794) who as a youth in the care of his father was with Captain James Cook on his second and third voyages. Doctor, explorer and botanist, he later became a revolutionary and writer. The genus Forstera commemorates both father and son, both doctor-botanists.

Engraving by Wegersc of Leipzig, courtesy of The Hunt Institute for Botanical Documentation, Carnegie Mellon University, Pittsburg and Ms Anita Karg.

FORSTER, Professor Johann Reinhold (1729–1798)

Major contributions to medicine, exploration, scholarship and civic life –

Minister of Religion, Surgeon, Naturalist, Explorer, Scholar

Countries of residence and civic and scientific contribution –

Prussia (Gdansk), England (Lancashire, London), Australia, Switzerland, Germany (Halle)

Scientific Name – Forstera spp.

FRANKENIUS, Professor Johan (1590–1661)

Major contributions to medicine, exploration, scholarship and civic life –

Doctor, Anatomist, Botanist

Countries of residence and civic and scientific contribution –

Sweden (Uppsala)

Scientific Name – Frankenia spp.

FUIREN, Dr Jorgen (1581–1628)

Major contributions to medicine, exploration, scholarship and civic life –

Physician, Botanist

Countries of residence and civic and scientific contribution –

Switzerland, Denmark (Copenhagen, Jutland), Sweden (Gotland)

Scientific Name – Fuirena spp.

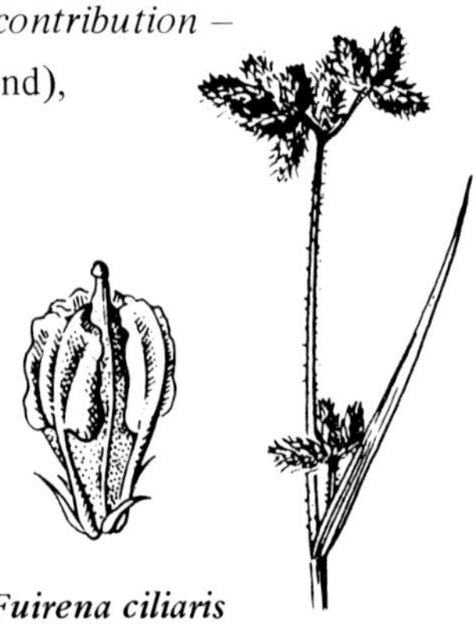

Fuirena ciliaris

GAERTNER, Professor Joseph (1732–1791)

Major contributions to medicine, exploration, scholarship and civic life –

Physician, Anatomist, Botanist

Countries of residence and civic and scientific contribution –

Germany (Tübingen, Göttingen, Wurttemburg), Russia (Leningrad), Ukraine, Holland (Leiden)

Scientific Name –

Gaertnera australiana (only one species of the 30 member genus in Australia)

GAHN, Dr Henrik (1747–1816)

Major contributions to medicine, exploration, scholarship and civic life –

Physician, Botanist, Military (Army), Teacher

Countries of residence and civic and scientific contribution –

Sweden (Uppsala, Stockholm), Holland, England, Scotland

Scientific Name – Gahnia spp.

GAIMARD, Surgeon Paul Joseph (1793–1858)

Major contributions to medicine, exploration, scholarship and civic life –

Naval Surgeon, Physician, Zoologist, Botanist, Collector

Countries of residence and civic and scientific contribution –

France (Paris), Australia (Western Australia)

Scientific Name – Gaimardia spp.

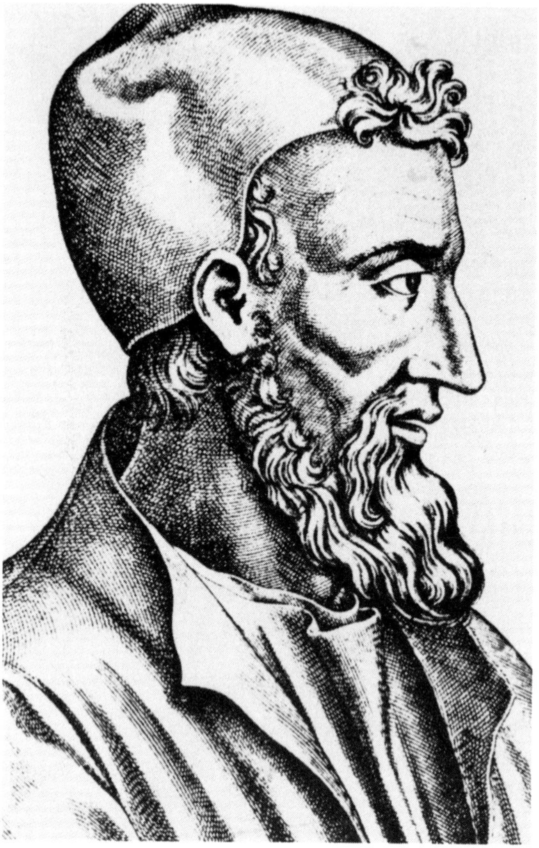

GALEN (130–200 A.D.) the Greek physician whose writings were unquestioned for more than one thousand years of Western medicine.

Several introduced species of Galenia are now endemic in Australia.

A modern artist's impression of one whose medical reputation is mixed – "both hero and villain".

GALEN, (130–200 A.D.

Major contributions to medicine, exploration, scholarship and civic life –
Physician, Physiologist

Countries of residence and civic and scientific contribution –
Greece, Cilicia (now Turkey in Asia Minor), Rome, Alexandria

Scientific Name – Galenia spp.

GARCIN, Surgeon Laurent (1683–1752)

Major contributions to medicine, exploration, scholarship and civic life –

Physician, Military Surgeon, Botanist, Collector, Explorer

Countries of residence and civic and scientific contribution –

France, Switzerland (Neuchatel), Holland (Leiden, Hulst), Portugal, Spain, India, Ceylon (now Sri Lanka), Indonesia

Scientific Name – *Garcinia* spp.

GARDEN, Dr Alexander (1728–1791)

Major contributions to medicine, exploration, scholarship and civic life –

Physician, Botanist, University Professor

Countries of residence and civic and scientific contribution –

United States of America (New York, Charleston), England (London)

Scientific Name – *Gardenia* spp.

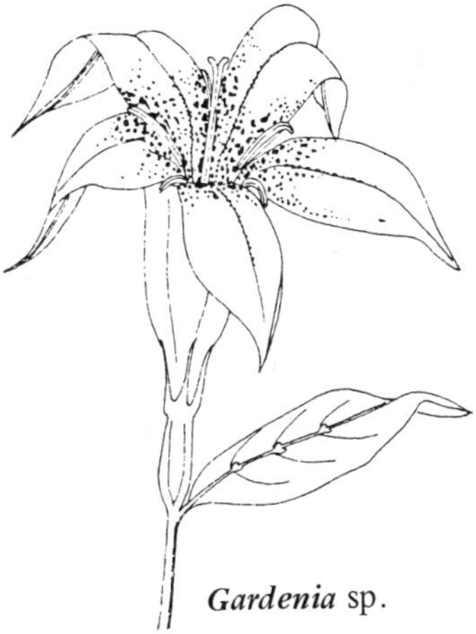

Gardenia sp.

GARNOT, Surgeon Prosper (1794–1838)

Major contributions to medicine, exploration, scholarship and civic life –

Naval Surgeon, Botanist, Explorer

Countries of residence and civic and scientific contribution –

France, Australia

Scientific Name –

Garnotia tortuosa
(a single species in Australia, found in North Queensland)

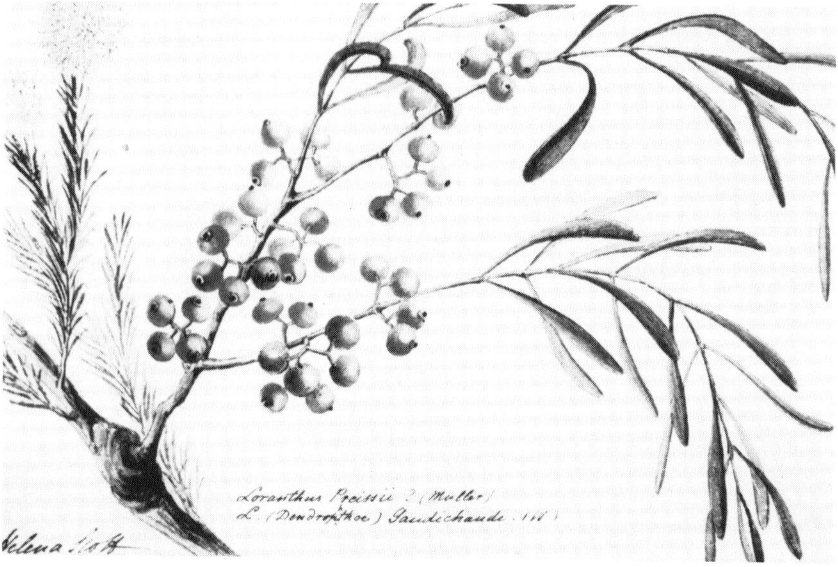

Professor Charles Gaudichaud-Beaupré (1789–1854) gave his name to Amyema gaudichaudii, formerly Loranthus gaudichaudii, a mistletoe of woody plants in many parts of Australia.

Gaudichaud-Beaupré was the apothecary-naturalist on board Freycinet's 'Uranie' and 'Physicienne' in its circumnavigation of the world 1817–1820 He collected when the expedition visited Port Jackson, travelling to Bathurst and the Blue Mountains.

This painting was produced by Miss Helena Scott in the period 1852-1883, at her home at Ash Island in the Lower Hunter River, N.S.W.

Reproduced by kind permission of The Mitchell Library, State Library of New South Wales, with acknowledgements.

GAUDICHAUD-BEAUPRÉ, Professor Charles (1789–1854)

Major contributions to medicine, exploration, scholarship and civic life –

Apothecary, Botanist, Explorer, Museum Patron,
Chief Naval Pharmacist

Countries of residence and civic and scientific contribution –

France (Paris), Falkland Islands (shipwrecked),
Australia (Western Australia, Port Jackson, Blue Mountains, Bathurst),
South Pacific, China (Canton)

Scientific Name – Carex gaudichaudiana

GAULTIER, Dr Jean-Francois (1708–1756)

Major contributions to medicine, exploration, scholarship and civic life –

Physician, Botanist

Countries of residence and civic and scientific contribution –

France, Canada

Scientific Name – Gaultheria spp.

GIBSON, Surgeon Alexander (1800–1867)

Major contributions to medicine, exploration, scholarship and civic life –

Surgeon, Botanist, Gardener, Forester

Countries of residence and civic and scientific contribution –

Scotland (Edinburgh), India (Bombay)

Scientific Name – Hibiscus gibsonii

GILBEE, Dr William (1825–1885)

Major contributions to medicine, exploration, scholarship and civic life –

Surgeon, Goldminer, University Examiner

Countries of residence and civic and scientific contribution –

Scotland (Edinburgh), Australia (Tasmania, Melbourne),
United States of America (California)

Scientific Name – *Gillbeea adenopetala*

GILRUTH, Professor John Anderson (1871–1937)

Major contributions to medicine, exploration, scholarship and civic life –

Veterinary Surgeon, Bacteriologist, Public Health Commissioner,
Public Administration

Countries of residence and civic and scientific contribution –

Scotland (Glasgow), New Zealand,
Australia (Melbourne, Darwin)

Scientific Name –
Gilruthia osbornii (a monotypic genus)

GRAHAM, Dr George (1828–1893)

Major contributions to medicine, exploration, scholarship and civic life –

Surgeon, Psychiatrist, Patron of Medical Societies,
University Lecturer

Countries of residence and civic and scientific contribution –

England (London), Australia (Adelaide, Melbourne)

Scientific Name – *Elaeocarpus grahamii*

GREEVES, Dr Augustus Frederick Adolphus (1805–1874)

Major contributions to medicine, exploration, scholarship and civic life –

Surgeon, Politician, Mayor of Melbourne, Businessman

Countries of residence and civic and scientific contribution –

England (Harrowgate), Australia (Melbourne)

Scientific Names –

Greevesia spp.
Millotia greevesii

GREW, Dr Nehemiah (1641–1712)

Major contributions to medicine, exploration, scholarship and civic life –

Physician, Botanist, Astronomer, Chemist

Countries of residence and civic and scientific contribution –

England (Warwick, London), Holland (Leiden)

Scientific Name – *Grewia* spp.

GRIFFITH, Dr William (1810–1845)

Major contributions to medicine, exploration, scholarship and civic life –

Surgeon, Physician, Botanist, Professor of Medical Botany, Gardener, Collector

Countries of residence and civic and scientific contribution –

England (London), Bhutan, India (Madras, Assam, Calcutta), Afghanistan, Malaysia (Malacca)

Scientific Name – *Parinari griffithianum*

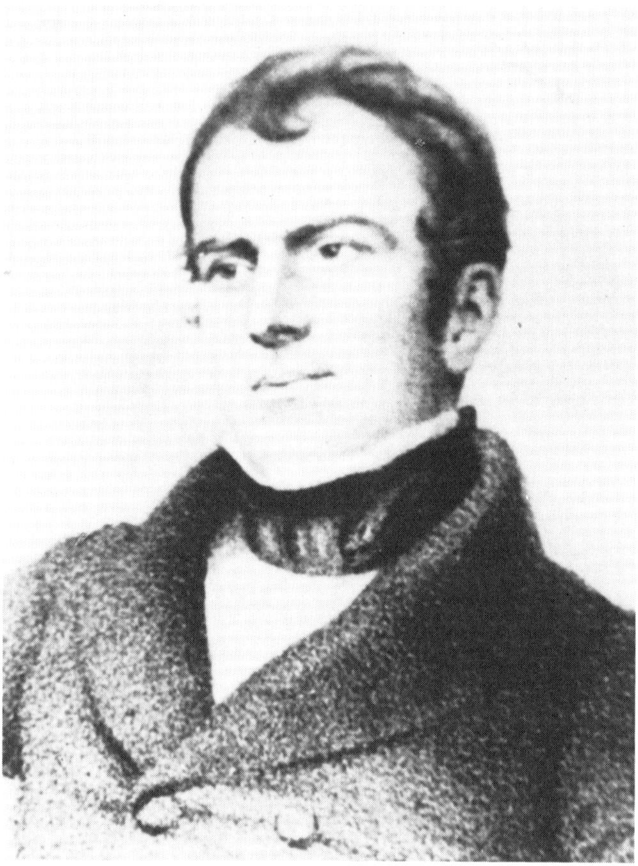

DR WILLIAM GRIFFITH (1810–1845)
Professor of Medical Botany, and
Physician to the East India Company in Madras and Calcutta.

He is commemorated in the northern Australian tree
Parinari griffithianum.

Portrait by kind permission of the Hunt Institute for
Botanical Documentation, Carnegie Mellon University,
Pittsburgh, with acknowledgements.

HAECKER, Dr Gottfried Renatus (1789–1864)

Major contributions to medicine, exploration, scholarship and civic life –

Apothecary, Botanist

Countries of residence and civic and scientific contribution –

Germany (Lübeck)

Scientific Name – Haeckeria spp.

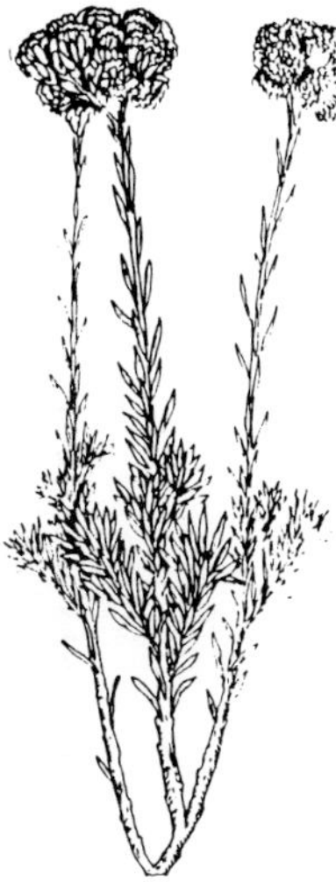

Haeckeria punctulata

HAIG, Dr William (1823–1893)

Major contributions to medicine, exploration, scholarship and civic life –

Surgeon, Physician, Surgeon Superintendent-Emigrant Ship, Public Health Officer, Magistrate, Pioneer, Collector, Military Surgeon

Countries of residence and civic and scientific contribution –

England, United States of America (Baltimore, New York), Australia (Melbourne)

Scientific Name – Helipterum haigii

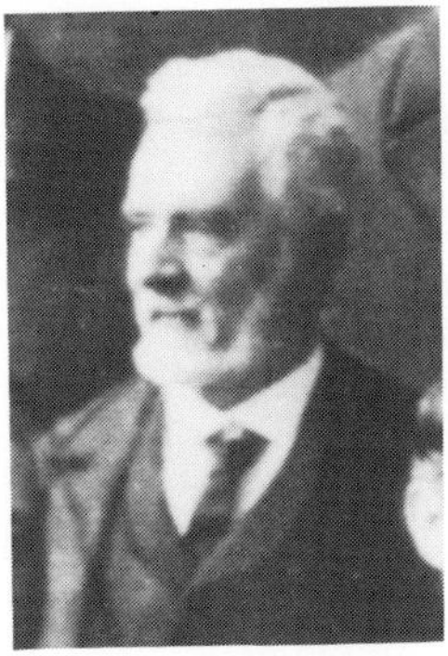

Dr WILLIAM HAIG (1823–1893) Military surgeon, surgeon-superintendent of emigrants, and collector. Haig's Everlasting, the sunray Helipterum haigii, is his memorial. Photo, taken at the Intercolonial Medical Congress held in Melbourne in 1889, courtesy of the Australian Medical Association (Victorian Branch).

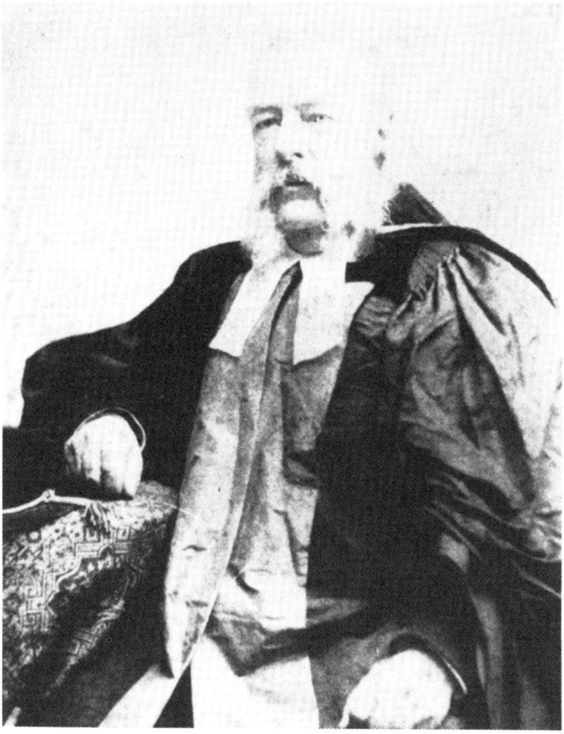

PROFESSOR GEORGE BRITTON HALFORD
(1824–1910)

A Founder of Australia's first medical school (in Melbourne). Foundation Professor of Physiology, Anatomy and Pathology, he later became Dean of the Faculty of Medicine at Melbourne University.

The Australian genus Halfordia commemorates his name.

HALFORD, Professor George Britton (1824–1910)

Major contributions to medicine, exploration, scholarship and civic life –

Physiologist, Physician, Surgeon, Anatomist,
Pathologist, Dean of Medicine

Countries of residence and civic and scientific contribution –

England (Liverpool, London),
Australia (Melbourne)

Scientific Name – *Halfordia* spp.

HAMPTON, Dr John Stephen (1809–1869)

Major contributions to medicine, exploration, scholarship and civic life –

Naval Surgeon, Doctor to Convicts, Governor

Countries of residence and civic and scientific contribution –

Scotland (Edinburgh), West Indies, Mexico,
England (Plymouth), Australia (Tasmania, Perth),
Canada

Scientific Name – *Astrotricha hamptonii*

HANNA, Dr William John (*b.* 1938)

Major contributions to medicine, exploration, scholarship and civic life –

Surgeon

Countries of residence and civic and scientific contribution –

Ireland (Belfast), Australia (Mudgee, Bendigo)

Scientific Name – *Dahlia bipinnata "Dr Bill Hanna"*

HARVEY, Professor William Henry (1811–1866)

Major contributions to medicine, exploration, scholarship and civic life –

Physiologist, Botanist, Explorer, Professor of Botany,
Colonial Treasurer (Cape of Good Hope)

Countries of residence and civic and scientific contribution –

Ireland (Dublin), South Africa (Cape Town), England,
United States of America, Australia (W.A., Tasmania, Sydney
(Victoria), South Pacific, South America

Scientific Names –

Harveya spp.
Sarcopetalum harveyanum

HEARN, Dr W.E. (*fl.* 1866, *died* 1893)

Major contributions to medicine, exploration, scholarship and civic life –

Doctor

Countries of residence and civic and scientific contribution –

Australia (Hamilton, Victoria, Western Australia)

Scientific Name – *Trichosanthes hearnii*

von HELMHOLTZ, Professor Hermann Ludwig Ferdinand (1821–1894)

Major contributions to medicine, exploration, scholarship and civic life –

Physiologist, Military Surgeon, Anatomist, Physicist, Chemist,
Inventor, Writer, Musicologist

Countries of residence and civic and scientific contribution –

Germany (Potsdam, Berlin, Koenigsberg, Bonn, Heidelberg)

Scientific Name – *Helmholtzia* spp.

HERNANDEZ, Dr Francisco (1514–1587)

Major contributions to medicine, exploration, scholarship and civic life –

Physician, Botanist, Naturalist

Countries of residence and civic and scientific contribution –

Spain (Toledo, Madrid), West Indies

Scientific Name – Hernandia spp.

HILLEBRAND, Dr Wilhelm (1821–1886)

Major contributions to medicine, exploration, scholarship and civic life –

Doctor, Botanist, Collector

Countries of residence and civic and scientific contribution –

Germany (Westfalen, Heidelberg), Hawaii, United States of America (California), Asia (Hong Kong), Indonesia (Java), Australia

Scientific Name – Phebalium hillebrandii

HIPPOCRATES (460 B.C. – 370 B.C.)

Major contributions to medicine, exploration, scholarship and civic life –

Physician, Medical Teacher, "Father of Medicine"

Countries of residence and civic and scientific contribution –

Greece (Kos)

Scientific Name –

Salacicratea spp.
(An anagram of two genera *Hippocratea* and *Salacia*)

HOGG, Dr Alison (*b.*

Major contributions to medicine, exploration, scholarship and civic life –

Doctor, Community Practitioner

Countries of residence and civic and scientific contribution –

Australia (Melbourne)

Scientific Name –

Dahlia bipinnata
"Dr Alison Hogg"

HOOKER, Sir Joseph Dalton (1817–1911)

Major contributions to medicine, exploration, scholarship and civic life –

Naval Surgeon, Botanist, Scientist,
Collector, Explorer, Geographer,
Writer, Scholar, Gardener

Countries of residence and civic and scientific contribution –

Scotland (Glasgow, Edinburgh),
England (London), Antarctica,
Australia (Tasmania, Sydney),
New Zealand, South America
(Tierra del Fuego, Falkland Islands),
India (Darjeeling, Himalayas),
Nepal, Syria, Africa (Morocco),
United States of America
(Colorado, Wyoming, Utah,
California)

Scientific Name – Olearia hookeri

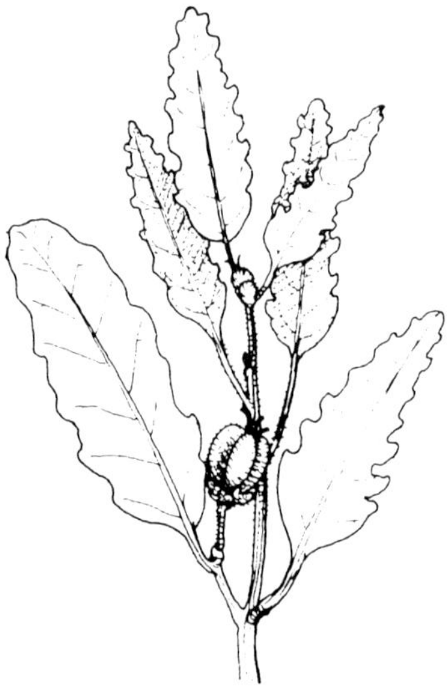

Adriana hookeri

HORNSTEDT, Dr Claes Frederick (1758–1809)

Major contributions to medicine, exploration, scholarship and civic life –

Doctor, Naturalist, Prisoner-of-War

Countries of residence and civic and scientific contribution –

Sweden (Linkoping), Finland (Helsinki)

Scientific Name –

Hornstedtia scottiana (syn. *Elettaria scottiana*)

HORSFIELD, Dr Thomas (1773–1859)

Major contributions to medicine, exploration, scholarship and civic life –

Doctor, Explorer, Botanist, Ornithologist,
Natural Historian, Museum Curator

Countries of residence and civic and scientific contribution –

United States of America (Pennsylvania),
Indonesia (Java, Sumatra),
England (London)

Scientific Name –

Horsfieldia australiana
(one species only in Australia, of this genus of some 80 species)

HOUSE, Dr Frederick Maurice (1865–1936)

Major contributions to medicine, exploration, scholarship and civic life –

Doctor, Naturalist, Magistrate, Ornithologist, Explorer,
Military Surgeon, Pastoralist

Countries of residence and civic and scientific contribution –

England (Alverstoke, London), Australia (Beverley, Katanning,
Derby, Gnowangerup, all in Western Australia), Egypt

Scientific Name – Eucalyptus houseana

HOUSTOUN, Dr William (1695–1733)

Major contributions to medicine, exploration, scholarship and civic life –

Doctor, Botanist, Collector

Countries of residence and civic and scientific contribution –

Scotland,
Central America

Scientific Name –

Ageratum houstonianum
(a native of South America, now naturalized and widespread in Queensland where it is known as "Blue Billygoat Weed")

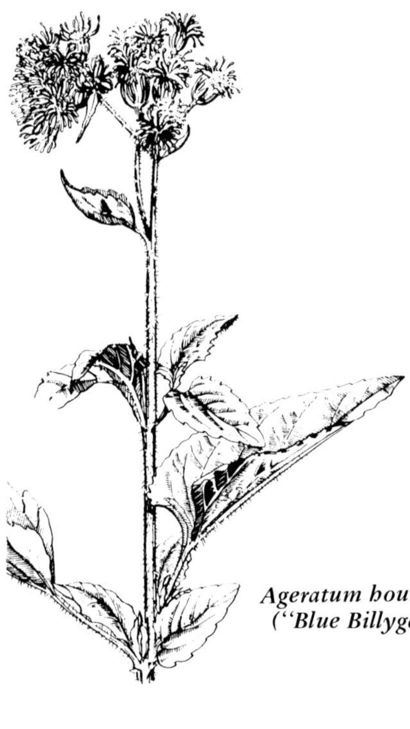

Ageratum houstonianum
("Blue Billygoat Weed")

HOWITT, Dr Godfrey (1800–1873)

Major contributions to medicine, exploration, scholarship and civic life –

Physician, Anthropologist, Explorer, Naturalist,
Medical Educator, Entomologist, Pastoralist,
University Councillor

Countries of residence and civic and scientific contribution –

England (Mansfield, Nottingham),
Australia (Melbourne)

Scientific Names –

Howittia trilocularis
(a monotypic genus)
Zygophyllum howittii

HUXLEY, Dr Thomas Henry (1825–1895)

Major contributions to medicine, exploration, scholarship and civic life –

Naval Surgeon, Botanist, Zoologist, Natural Historian,
Anthropologist, Scholar, Philosopher, Writer

Countries of residence and civic and scientific contribution –

England (London),
Australia (Sydney, Melbourne, Tasmania, Darling Downs),
New Guinea

Scientific Name –

Huxleya linifolia
(a monotypic genus found in the Northern Territory)

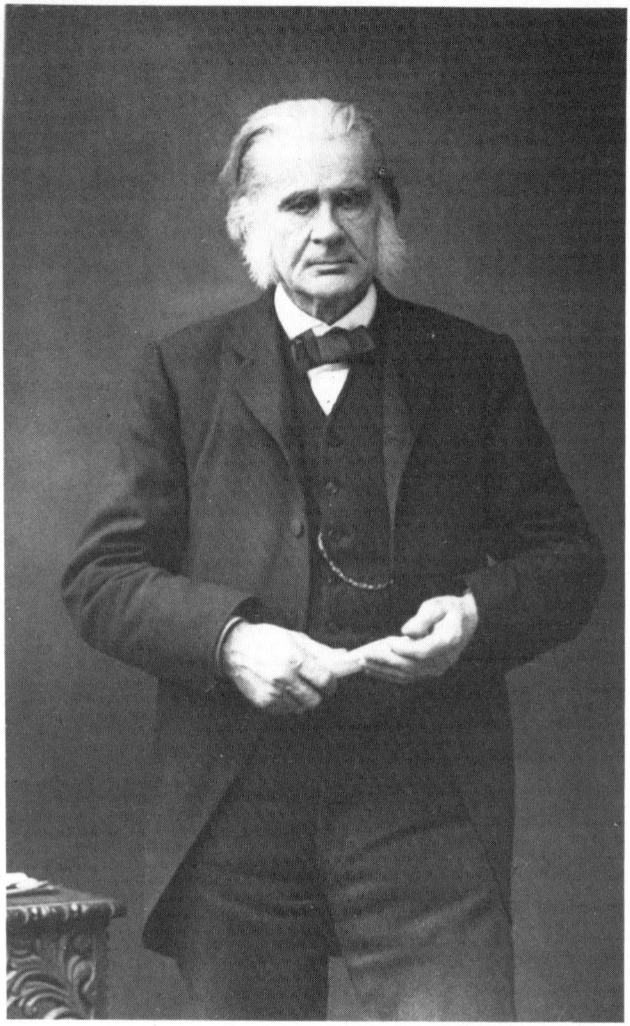

DR THOMAS HENRY HUXLEY (1825–1895)

President of the Royal Society of London, naval surgeon, scholar, philosopher and natural historian.
As surgeon and naturalist on board HMS 'Rattlesnake' he spent three years in Australia, writing later that his 'scientific career practically commenced ... in Australian seas ... the strongest ties of my life were found in Sydney'.
The Northern Territory genus, Huxleya, commemorates his name.

IFFLA, Dr Solomon (1821–1887)

Major contributions to medicine, exploration, scholarship and civic life –

Doctor, Politician, Psychiatrist, Natural Historian

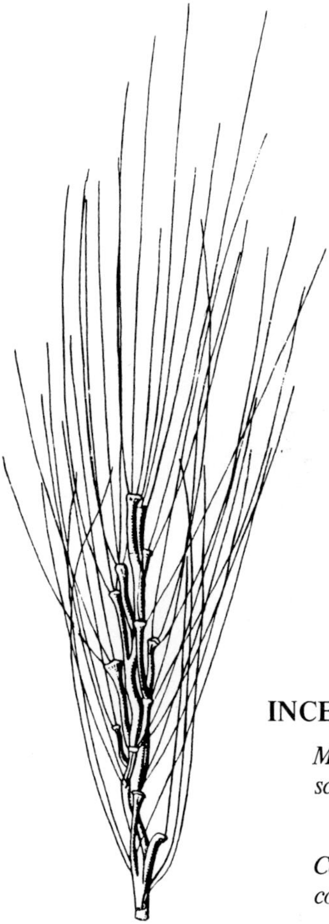

Countries of residence and civic and scientific contribution –

Jamaica, United States of America (Philadelphia), Scotland (Glasgow), Australia (Adelaide, Melbourne, Wood's Point)

Scientific Name – Flindersia ifflaiana

IMPERATO, Ferrante (1550–1625)

Major contributions to medicine, exploration, scholarship and civic life –

Apothecary, Botanist, Gardener, Palaeontologist

Countries of residence and civic and scientific contribution –

Italy (Naples)

Scientific Name –

Imperata cylindrica
(one species only in Australia)

INCE, Dr Walter Holinshed (1895–1907)

Major contributions to medicine, exploration, scholarship and civic life –

Pharmacist, Medical Chemist

Countries of residence and civic and scientific contribution –

England (London), West Indies (Trinidad)

Scientific Name – Acacia inceae

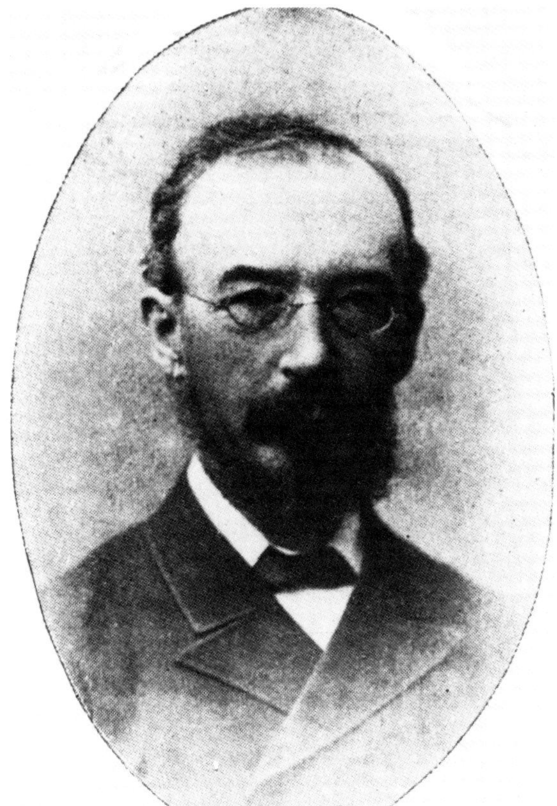

DR JAMES JAMIESON MD
(1840–1916)

Pioneer medical teacher at the University of Melbourne. The beautiful morrison, Verticordia jamiesonii, commemorates his name. Photo by Johnstone and O'Shannessy, courtesy of the Brownless Memorial Supplement (to 'Alma Mater'), University of Melbourne, September 1898.

JAMIESON, Dr James (1840–1916)

Major contributions to medicine, exploration, scholarship and civic life –

Ship's Surgeon, Physician, Obstetrician, Paediatrician,
Public Health Officer, Medical Educator, Publicist

Countries of residence and civic and scientific contribution –

Scotland (Glasgow), Australia (Warrnambool, Melbourne)

Scientific Name – Verticordia jamiesonii

JEANNERETT, Dr Henry (1802–1886)

Major contributions to medicine, exploration, scholarship and civic life –

Surgeon, Physician, Dentist, Botanist,
Superintendent of Aborigines

Countries of residence and civic and scientific contribution –

England (Oxford, London), Scotland (Edinburgh),
Australia (Sydney, Port Arthur, Flinder's Island)

Scientific Name – Jeannerettia spp.

JOHNSON, Dr Thomas (? – 1644)

Major contributions to medicine, exploration, scholarship and civic life –

Apothecary, Physician, Gardener, Botanist

Country of residence and civic and scientific contribution –

England (Lincolnshire, London)

Scientific Name – Johnsonia spp.

JONES, Sir Philip Sydney (1836–1918)

Major contributions to medicine, exploration, scholarship and civic life –

Physician, Surgeon, Medical Educator,
University Vice-Chancellor,
Philanthropist, Churchman

Country of residence and civic and scientific contribution –

Australia (Sydney)

Scientific Name – Acacia jonesii

de JUSSIEU, Dr Bernard (1699–1777)

Major contributions to medicine, exploration, scholarship and civic life –

Botanist, Doctor

Country of residence and civic and scientific contribution –

France (Paris)

Scientific Name –

Jussiaea spp.
(now syn. with *Ludwigia*)

KENNY, Sister Elizabeth (1880–1952)

Major contributions to medicine, exploration, scholarship and civic life –

Nurse, Army Nurse,
Poliomyelitis – Campaigner/Therapist,
Honorary M.D., Physical Therapist

Countries of residence and civic and scientific contribution –

Australia (Queensland),
United States of America (Minnesota, New York)

Scientific Names –

Dahlia bipinnata "Sister Kenny"
Rosa sp. ("Sister Kenny") (A Floribunda Rose)

KERAUDREN, Dr Pierre Francois (1769–1851)

Major contributions to medicine, exploration, scholarship and civic life –

Naval Surgeon, Physician, Naturalist

Countries of residence and civic and scientific contribution –

France (Brittany)

Scientific Name – *Keraudrenia* spp.

KESTEVEN, Dr Hereward Leighton (1881–1964)

Major contributions to medicine, exploration, scholarship and civic life –

Doctor, Malacologist, Zoologist, Botanist, Anatomist,
Farmer, Writer, Industrial Medical Officer

Countries of residence and civic and scientific contribution –

Fiji (Levuka), Australia (Brisbane, Sydney, Gin Gin, Gladstone,
Bulahdelah, Cooktown, Palmwoods, Maroochydore)

Scientific Name – *Dendrobium kestevenii*

KOENIG, Dr Johann Gerhard (1728–1785)

Major contributions to medicine, exploration, scholarship and civic life –

Doctor, Missionary, Botanist, Pharmacist, Collector

Countries of residence and civic and scientific contribution –

Latvia, Sweden, Denmark, South Africa (Cape of Good Hope), India, Siam, Ceylon (Sri Lanka), Iceland

Scientific Name – *Scaevola koenigii*

KREYSIG, Dr Friedrich Ludwig (1770–1839)

Major contributions to medicine, exploration, scholarship and civic life –

Physician

Countries of residence and civic and scientific contribution –

Germany (Dresden)

Scientific Name –

Kreysigia multiflora (a monotypic genus)

KRUSE, John (1822–1895)

Major contributions to medicine, exploration, scholarship and civic life –

Pharmacist, Chemist

Countries of residence and civic and scientific contribution –

Germany (Emden, Goettingen),
England (London),
Australia

Scientific Name –

Eucalyptus kruseana

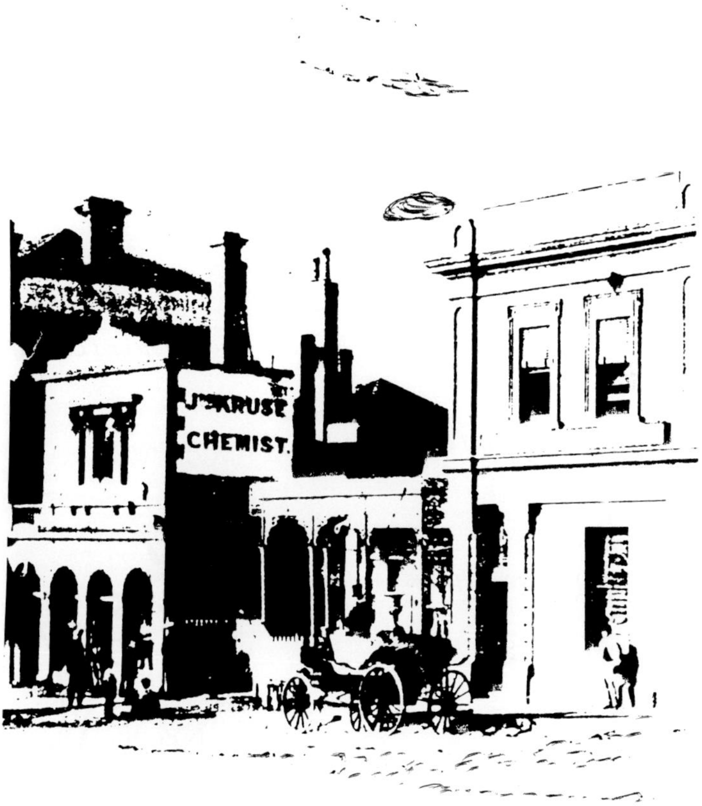

The pharmacy of JOHN KRUSE, Russell Street, Melbourne, circa 1866

Pharmaceutical chemist and medical scientist, John Kruse (1822–1895) was a founder of the Pharmaceutical Society of Victoria and Lecturer in Materia Medica and Botany at the School (later College) of Pharmacy.

Photo, courtesy of the Kruse family and of the Victorian College of Pharmacy, Melbourne, with grateful acknowledgements.

KUNZE, Professor Gustav (1793–1851)

Major contributions to medicine, exploration, scholarship and civic life –
Physician, Botanist, Professor of Medicine

Countries of residence and civic and scientific contribution –
Germany (Leipzig)

Scientific Name – *Kunzea* spp.

KYLLING, Peter Lauridson (*c.* 1640–1696)

Major contributions to medicine, exploration, scholarship and civic life –
Apothecary, Botanist

Countries of residence and civic and scientific contribution –
Denmark

Scientific Name –
Kyllinga spp. (syn. *Cyperus*)

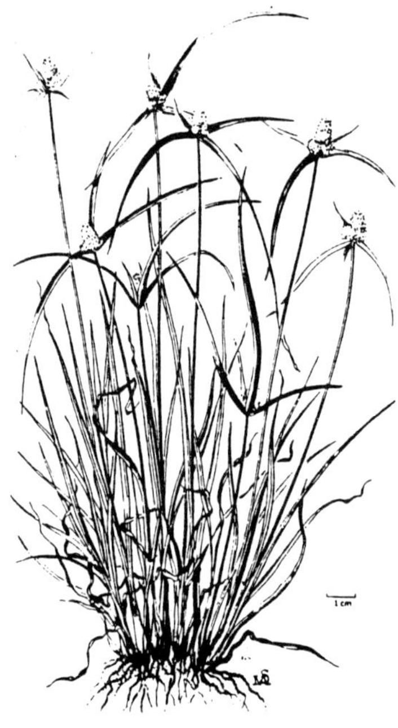

Kyllinga Weed, or Cyperus sesquitflorus, a sedge of damp places in north-eastern Australia.

The genus Kyllinga (syn. Cyperus) commemorates PETER KYLLING (c. 1640–1696), a Danish apothecary.

(Illustration courtesy of Dr Robert Johnson and the artist, Mr Will Smith.)

van der LAAN, Dr Pieter Adrianus (*fl.* 1880)

Major contributions to medicine, exploration, scholarship and civic life –

Physician, Ophthalmologist

Countries of residence and civic and scientific contribution –

Holland (Utrecht), Spain

Scientific Name – Eremophila laanii

de LAGUNA, Dr Andreas (1499–1560)

Major contributions to medicine, exploration, scholarship and civic life –

Physician, Anatomist, Physiologist, Writer, Botanist

Countries of residence and civic and scientific contribution –

Spain (Segovia), Italy (Rome), France (Metz)

Scientific Name –

Lagunaria patersonii
(a monotypic genus)

LANG, Dr Patrick Henry (1875–1947)

Major contributions to medicine, exploration, scholarship and civic life –

Military Surgeon, Doctor, Pastoralist, Horticulturalist

Countries of residence and civic and scientific contribution –

Scotland (Selkirk), Australia (Ararat, Camperdown, Lismore in Victoria), England (London), South Africa, France (Rouen)

Scientific Name – Eucalyptus langii

LATZ, Peter (*b.* 1942)

Major contributions to medicine, exploration, scholarship and civic life –
Botanist, Medical Anthropologist

Countries of residence and civic and scientific contribution –
Australia (Alice Springs)

Scientific Name – Aristida latzii

LAURENTI, Professor Mario Antonio

Major contributions to medicine, exploration, scholarship and civic life –
Physician, Professor of Medicine

Countries of residence and civic and scientific contribution –
Italy (Bologna)

Scientific Name –
Laurentia (Tr. *Isotoma*)

LAUTERER, Dr Joseph (1848–1911)

Major contributions to medicine, exploration, scholarship and civic life –
Military Surgeon, Doctor, Botanist, Zoologist,
Writer, Phytochemist

Countries of residence and civic and scientific contribution –
Germany (Freiburg, Karlsruhe),
Australia (Blue Mountains, Brisbane)

Scientific Name – Arytera lautereriana

LAVATER, Dr Johann Caspar (1741–1801)

Major contributions to medicine, exploration, scholarship and civic life –

Physiognomist, Naturalist, Pastor, Poet-Mystic

Countries of residence and civic and scientific contributions –

Switzerland (Zurich)

Scientific Name – *Lavatera* spp.

LAWSON, Dr Isaac (? – ? 1747)

Major contributions to medicine, exploration, scholarship and civic life –

Military Physician, Botanist, Collector

Countries of residence and civic and scientific contribution –

Scotland, Holland (Leiden, Oosterhout)

Scientific Name – *Lawsonia* spp.

LEDWARD, Dr Colin Prentice (1903–1963)

Major contributions to medicine, exploration, scholarship and civic life –

Doctor, Botanist, Zoologist, Lepidopterist

Countries of residence and civic and scientific contribution –

England (London), Australia (Canungra, Cloncurry, Burleigh Heads)

Scientific Name – *Acianthus ledwardii*

LEERS, Johann Georg Daniel (1727–1774)

Major contributions to medicine, exploration, scholarship and civic life –

Apothecary, Botanist

Countries of residence and civic and scientific contribution –

Germany (Herborn)

Scientific Name –

Leersia australis (One species only of the genus is in Australia)

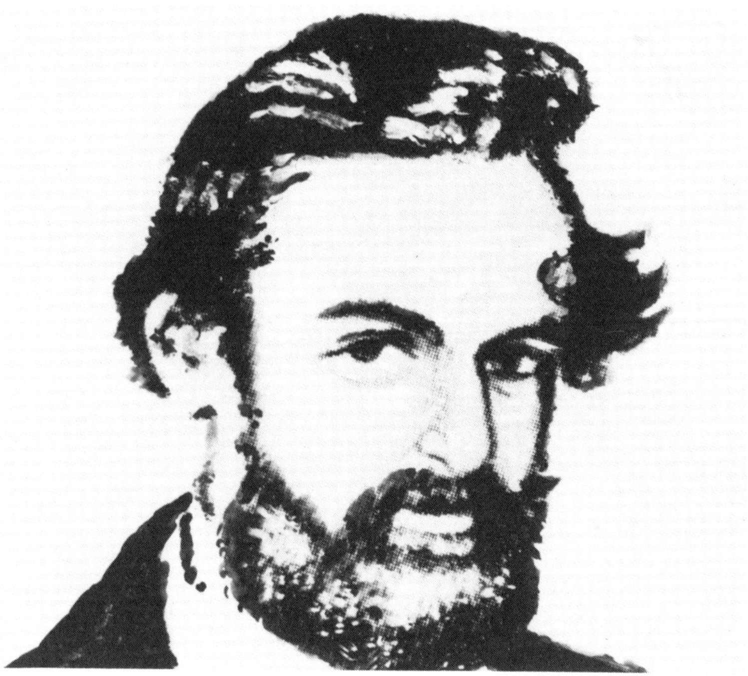

Dr LUDWIG LEICHHARDT (1813–1848), enigmatic explorer and botanist – the colonial title "Doctor" fitted well with his application to studies of biology and natural history in its many forms. Several dozen plants bear his name, including the several species within the genus Leichhardtia.

LEICHHARDT, Dr Friedrich Wilhelm Ludwig (1813–1848)

Major contributions to medicine, exploration, scholarship and civic life –

(Doctor), Explorer, Botanist, Geologist

Countries of residence and civic and scientific contribution –

Germany (Berlin, Gottingen), England (Gloucestershire, London), Australia (Sydney, Hunter River, Queensland, Northern Territory)

Scientific Names –

Leichhardtia spp.
Duboisia leichhardtii

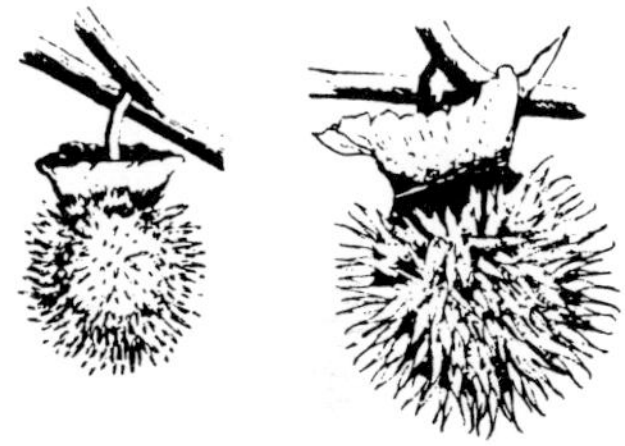

Datura leichbardtii

LESCHENAULT de la Tour, Surgeon Jean-Baptiste Louis-Claude-Theodore (1773–1826)

Major contributions to medicine, exploration, scholarship and civic life –

Surgeon, Naval Surgeon, Naturalist

Countries of residence and civic and scientific contribution –

France (Chalons-Sur-Saone, Paris), Australia (W.A.,S.A., Tasmania, Sydney), Java, Africa (Cape of Good Hope, Cape Verde Island), Madagascar, India (Pondicherry, Coimbetore), Ceylon (Sri Lanka), U.S.A. (Philadelphia), South America (French Guyana, Brazil)

Scientific Name – Lechenaultia spp.

LEVIER, Dr Emilio (1839–1911)

Major contributions to medicine, exploration, scholarship and civic life –

Physician, Botanist, Collector

Countries of residence and civic and scientific contribution –

Switzerland (Berne), France, Spain, Italy (Florence, Tuscany)

Scientific Name –

Levieria acuminata (sole species in Australia)

LEWELLIN, Dr Henry Hill (1818–1886)

Major contributions to medicine, exploration, scholarship and civic life –

Surgeon

Countries of residence and civic and scientific contribution –

India (Calcutta), England (London), Australia (Melbourne)

Scientific Name –

Dicrastylis lewellinii

LHOTSKY, Dr Johann (1800–*c.* 1861)

Major contributions to medicine, exploration, scholarship and civic life –

Surgeon, Explorer, Natural Historian, Zoologist, Linguist and Anthropologist, Botanist, Geologist, Writer, Collector and Curator

Countries of residence and civic and scientific contribution –

Austria (Vienna), Germany (Berlin), Hungary (Prague), Brazil, Australia (Sydney, Australian Alps, Queanbeyan, Tasmania), South Pacific

Scientific Name – *Lhotskya* spp.

von LINDERN, Dr Franz Balthasar (1682–1755)

Major contributions to medicine, exploration, scholarship and civic life –

Doctor, Botanist

Countries of residence and civic and scientific contribution –

France (Strasbourg)

Scientific Name – *Lindernia* spp.

LINNAEUS, Professor Carolus (von Linne, Carl)(1707–1778)

Major contributions to medicine, exploration, scholarship and civic life –

Doctor, Botanist, Zoologist, Explorer, "Father of Modern Botany", Professor of Medicine and Botany

Countries of residence and civic and scientific contribution –

Sweden (Stockholm, Uppsala), Lapland, Holland (Hartecamp)

Scientific Name – Indigofera linnaei

LINOCIER, Dr Geoffroi

Major contributions to medicine, exploration, scholarship and civic life –

Doctor

Countries of residence and civic and scientific contribution –

France

Scientific Name – Linociera spp.

deL'OBEL, Dr Mathias (1538–1616)

Major contributions to medicine, exploration, scholarship and civic life –

Physician, Botanist, Gardener

Countries of residence and civic and scientific contribution –

France (Lille, Montpellier), Belgium, England (London), Denmark

Scientific Name – Lobelia spp.

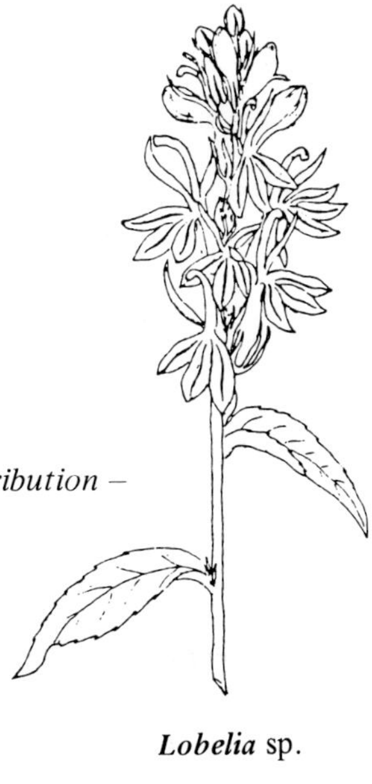

Lobelia sp.

LONGET (*fl.* 1866)

Major contributions to medicine, exploration, scholarship and civic life –

Physician

Countries of residence and civic and scientific contribution –

France

Scientific Name – Longetia spp. (Trans. *Austrobuxus*)

LUCAS, Professor Arthur Henry Shakespeare (1853–1936)

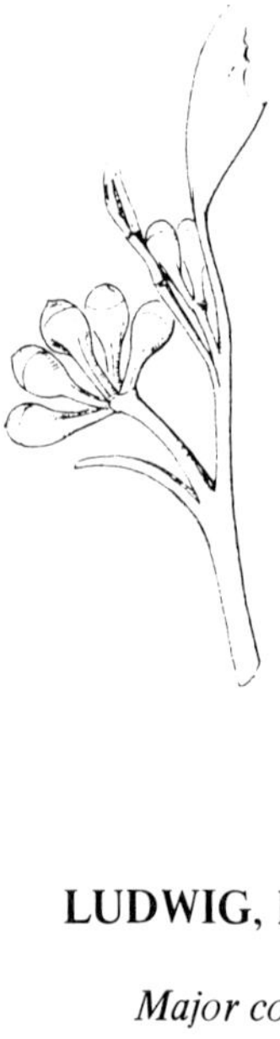

Major contributions to medicine, exploration, scholarship and civic life –

Medical Student, Botanist, Teacher & Headmaster, Writer, Natural Historian, University Lecturer

Countries of residence and civic and scientific contribution –

England (Oxford, Cambridge, London)
Australia (Melbourne, Sydney, Tasmania, Lord Howe Island, Queensland)

Scientific Name – Eucalyptus lucasii

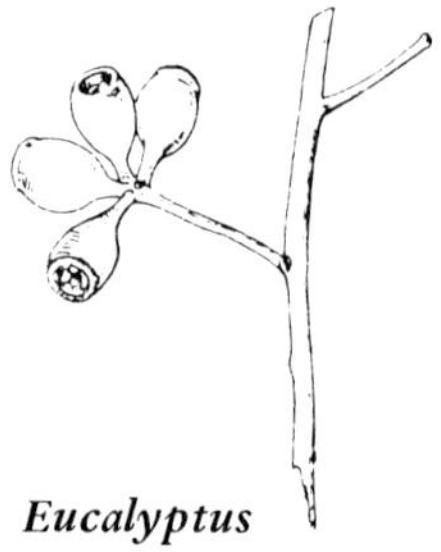

Eucalyptus lucasii

LUDWIG, Professor Christian Gottlieb (1709–1773)

Major contributions to medicine, exploration, scholarship and civic life –

Physician, Botanist, Professor of Medicine

Countries of residence and civic and scientific contribution –

Germany (Schlesion, Leipzig), Africa

Scientific Name – Ludwigia spp.

MACADAM, Dr John (1827–1865)

Major contributions to medicine, exploration, scholarship and civic life –

Doctor, Chemist, Politician, Public Health Officer, Postmaster-General (Victoria), University Lecturer

Countries of residence and civic and scientific contribution –

Scotland (Glasgow), Australia (Melbourne, Castlemaine)

Scientific Name – Macadamia spp.

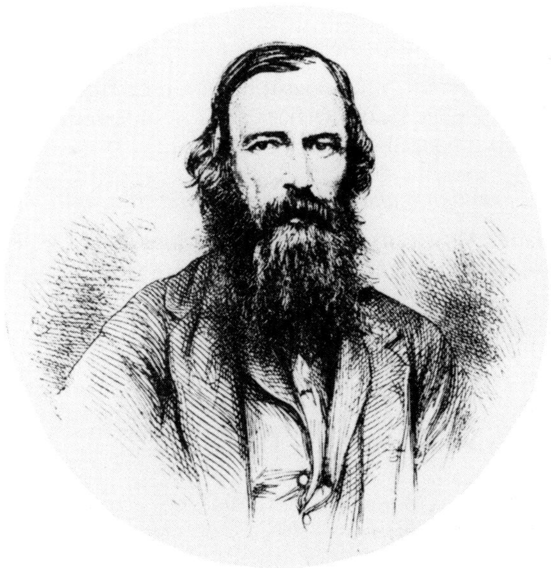

Mr JOHN MacGILLIVRAY
(1822–1867)

Medical student, explorer, collector and natural historian. Portrait engraving from 'Good Words'. Courtesy of Proceedings of the Australasian Association for the Advancement of Science, 1909.

MacGILLIVRAY, John (1822–1867)

Major contributions to medicine, exploration, scholarship and civic life –

Medical Student, Botanist, Explorer, Naturalist, Collector

Countries of residence and civic and scientific contribution –

Scotland (Aberdeen), South Pacific, Australia (Sydney, Queensland, Cape York, Lord Howe Island, Northern Territory)

Scientific Name – Nothopanax macgillivrayi

MacGREGOR, Sir William (1846–1919)

Major contributions to medicine, exploration, scholarship and civic life –

Doctor, Governor, Ethnologist, Explorer, Natural Historian, Collector, Public Health Officer, Civil Administrator, University Chancellor, Priory Councillor

Countries of residence and civic and scientific contribution –

Scotland (Aberdeen), Seychelles, Mauritius, New Guinea, Lagos, Newfoundland, Fiji, Australia (Brisbane)

Scientific Name – Danthonia macgregori

MACREDIE, Mr William (1813–1891)

Major contributions to medicine, exploration, scholarship and civic life –

Medical Administrator, Philanthropist

Countries of residence and civic and scientific contribution –

Scotland, Trinidad, Australia (Melbourne)

Scientific Name – Microcorys macrediana

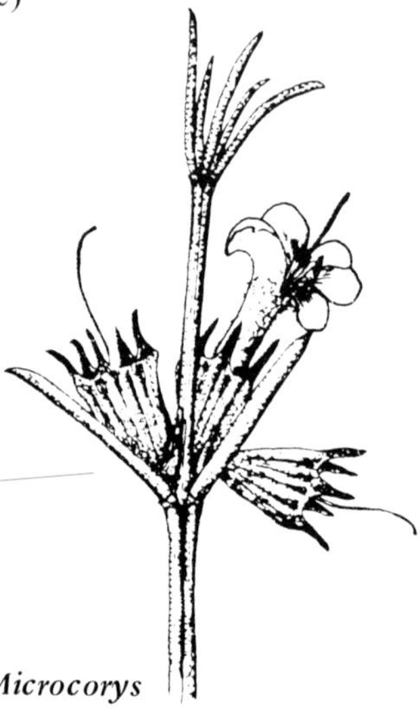

Microcorys macrediana

MARKS, Dr Charles Ferdinand Snr. (1852–1941)

Major contributions to medicine, exploration, scholarship and civic life –

Surgeon, Military Surgeon, Parliamentarian

Countries of residence and civic and scientific contribution –

Ireland (Galway), Australia (Brisbane)

Scientific Name – Cassia marksiana

MARTIN, Dr James (*fl.* 1863)

Major contributions to medicine, exploration, scholarship and civic life –

Doctor, Botanist, Explorer, Surveyor

Countries of residence and civic and scientific contribution –

Australia (Western Australia)

Scientific Name – Psoralea martinii

MAUND, Dr John (1823–1858)

Major contributions to medicine, exploration, scholarship and civic life –

Surgeon, Physician, Apothecary, Obstetrician,
Analytical Chemist, Hospital Patron, Public Health Officer

Countries of residence and civic and scientific contribution –

Scotland (Glasgow), England (Worcestershire),
Australia (Melbourne)

Scientific Name

Maundia triglochinoides
(a monotypic genus of water plant found in southern Queensland)

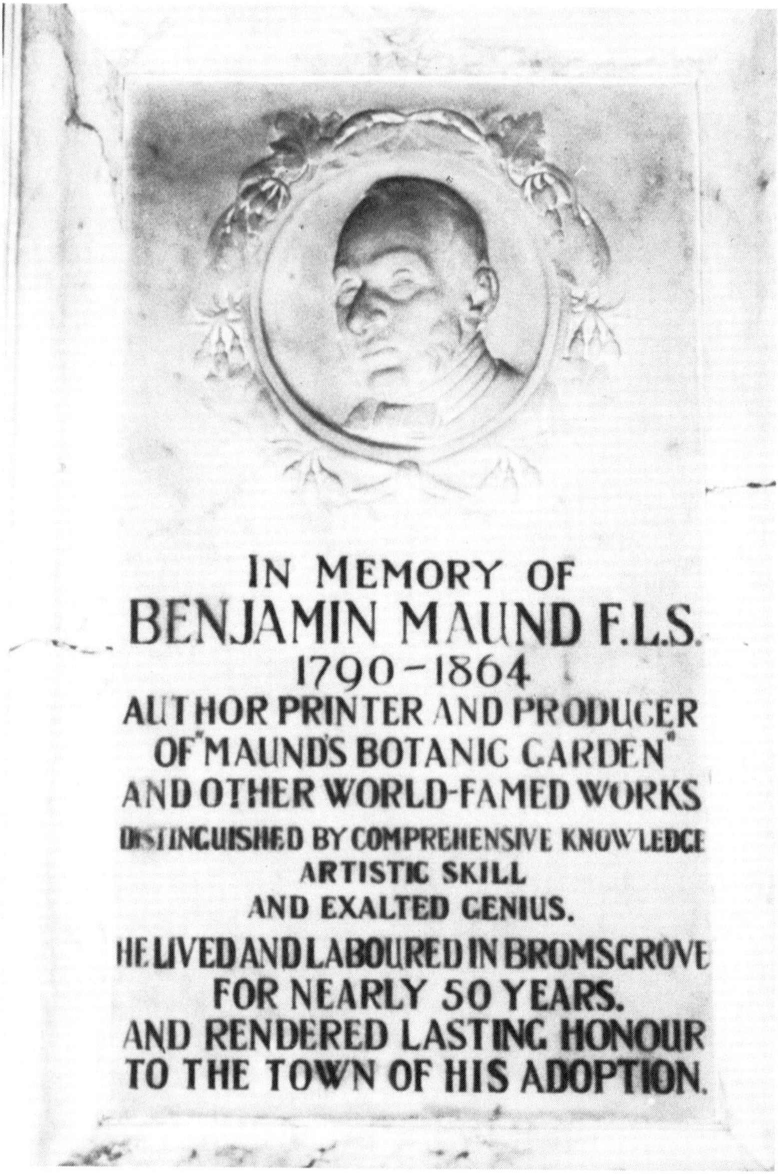

The plaque to Benjamin Maund (1790–1864), apothecary and botanist and father of Dr John Maund (1823–1858) of Melbourne. Bromsgrove Church, Worcestershire, England. Photo courtesy of Canon John Mushen, Rector.

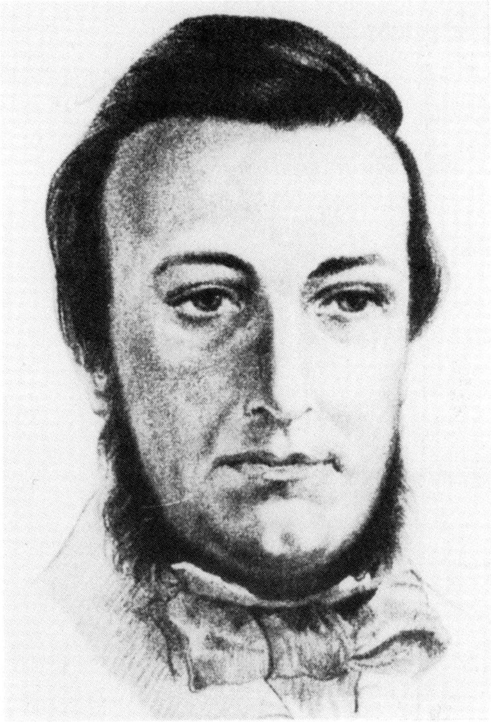

***Dr JOHN MAUND (1823–1858),** obstetrician and founder of The Royal Women's Hospital, Melbourne.*

The genus Maundia was named after him by Ferdinand von Mueller, at the time of the young obstetrician's death in 1858.

Photo courtesy of C.E. Sayers and The Royal Women's Hospital, Melbourne, with acknowledgements.

McCREA, Dr William (1814–1899)

Major contributions to medicine, exploration, scholarship and civic life –

Naval Surgeon, Surgeon – Department of Convicts,
Medical Administrator, Magistrate, Public Health Officer

Countries of residence and civic and scientific contribution –

Ireland (County Tyrone), England (London), North America,
North Africa, Australia (Tasmania, Melbourne)

Scientific Name – Xylopia maccreai

MEISSNER, Professor Carl Friedrich (1800–1874) (In his early years he spelt his patronymic "Meisner")

Major contributions to medicine, exploration, scholarship and civic life –

Physician, Botanist, Taxonomist, Writer, Professor of Botany

Countries of residence and civic and scientific contribution –

Switzerland (Berne, Basle)

Scientific Name – Acacia meissneri

MENKE, Dr Carl Theodor (1791–1861)

Major contributions to medicine, exploration, scholarship and civic life –

Physician, Botanist

Countries of residence and civic and scientific contribution –

Germany (Pyrmont)

Scientific Name – Menkea spp.

MENZIES, Surgeon Archibald (1754–1842)

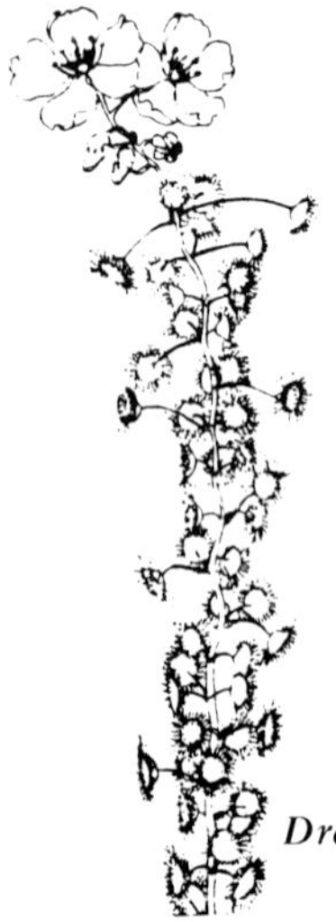

Major contributions to medicine, exploration, scholarship and civic life –

Naval Surgeon, Botanist, Explorer, Zoologist, Diarist, Gardener, Collector

Countries of residence and civic and scientific contribution –

Scotland (Perthshire), England (London), Australia (Western Australia), South Africa (Cape of Good Hope), China, Hawaii, West Indes, New Zealand, United States of America (California)

Scientific Name – Banksia menziesii

Drosera menziesii

MESSERSCHMID, Dr Daniel Gottlieb (1682–1735)

Major contributions to medicine, exploration, scholarship and civic life –

Physician, Botanist

Countries of residence and civic and scientific contribution –

Germany (Gdansk), Russia (Leningrad)

Scientific Name – *Messerschmidia argentea* (syn. *Argusia argentea* – sole species in Australia)

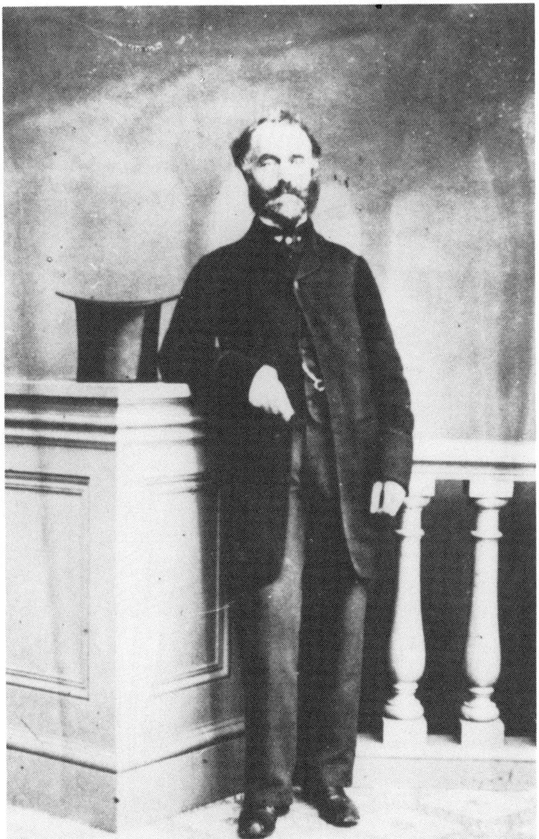

Surgeon Joseph Milligan (1807–1883). Botanist, ethnologist and collector, of Tasmania.

Photo (Carte de Visite) by L. Birnstinol of Hobart, 1862, courtesy of State Library of Tasmania.

MILLIGAN, Surgeon Joseph (1807–1883)

Major contributions to medicine, exploration, scholarship and civic life –
Surgeon, Botanist, Collector, Ethnologist, Natural Historian

Countries of residence and civic and scientific contribution –
Scotland (Dumfriesshire), Australia (Tasmania)

Scientific Names –

Milligania spp.
Pimelea milliganii

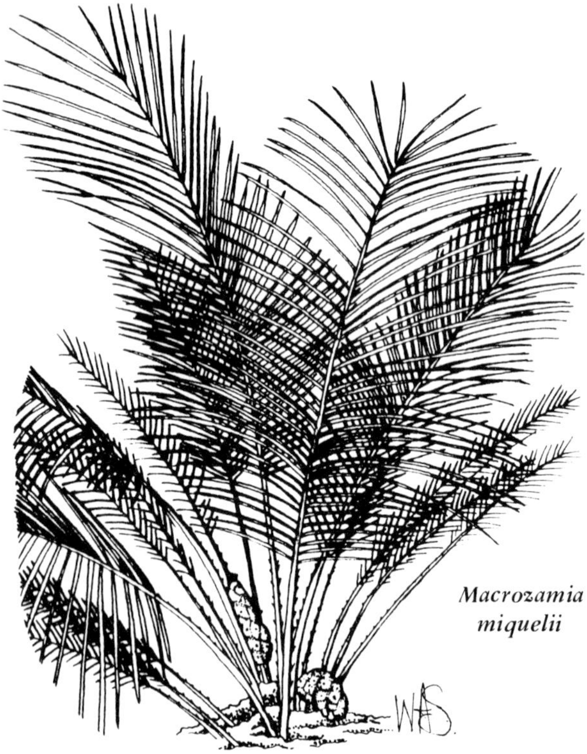

Macrozamia miquelii

MIQUEL, Professor Friedrich Anton Wilhelm (1811–1871)

Major contributions to medicine, exploration, scholarship and civic life –
Physician, Botanist, Gardener, Professor of Botany

Countries of residence and civic and scientific contribution –
Germany (Hanover) Holland (Utrecht, Rotterdam, Leiden)

Scientific Name – Grevillea miqueliana

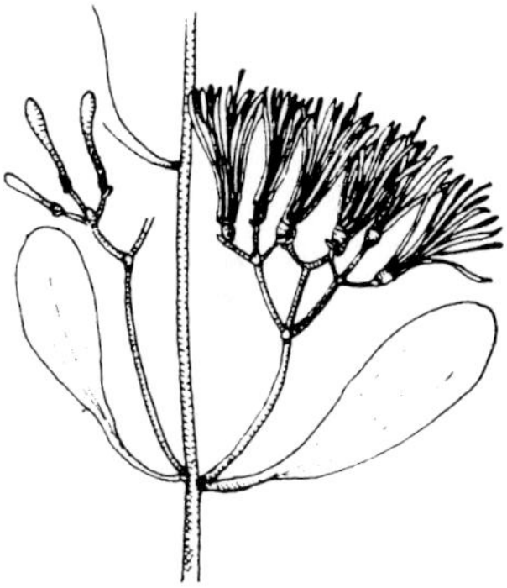

Amyema miquelii

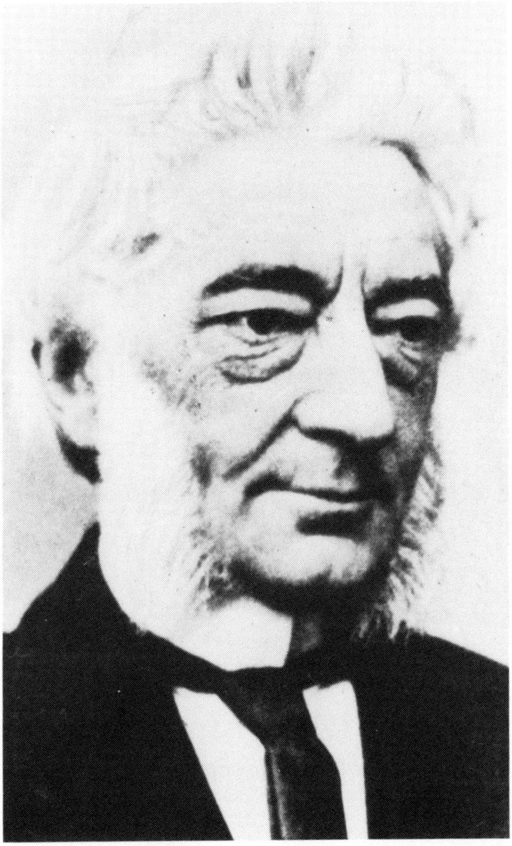

Professor Friedrich Anton Wilhelm Miquel (1811-1871), Dutch botanist and physician, whose name is recorded in an Australian cycad and a Grevillea.

Courtesy of The Rijksherbarium, Leiden, and Professor C.A. Kalkman.

MORGAN, Hugh (*fl.* 1540–1576)

Major contributions to medicine, exploration, scholarship and civic life –
Apothecary, Gardener

Country of residence and civic and scientific contribution –
England (London)

Scientific Name – *Morgania* spp.

MOTHERWELL, Dr James (*fl.* 1870)

Major contributions to medicine, exploration, scholarship and civic life –
Doctor, Patron of Science

Country of residence and civic and scientific contribution –
Australia (Melbourne)

Scientific Name –
Motherwellia haplosciadea (a monotypic genus)

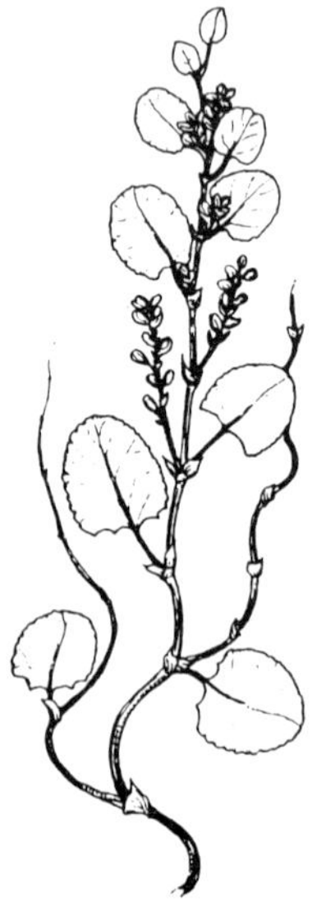

Muehlenbeckia adpressa

MUEHLENBECK, Dr Heinrich Gustav (1798–1845)

Major contributions to medicine, exploration, scholarship and civic life –

Physician, Botanist

Countries of residence and civic and scientific contribution –

France (St Marie-Aux-Mines, Paris),
Germany (Muhlhausen, Gebweiler)

Scientific Name – Muehlenbeckia spp.

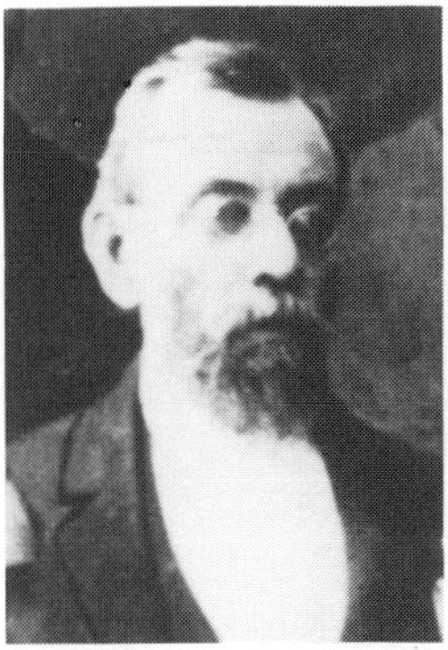

BARON FERDINAND JAKOB von MUELLER (1825–1896)

Great botanist, pharmacist and patron of Australian science.

Photo, at the Intercolonial Medical Congress held in Melbourne in 1889. Courtesy of the Victorian Branch of the Australian Medical Association, and Mr Ron Hastings.

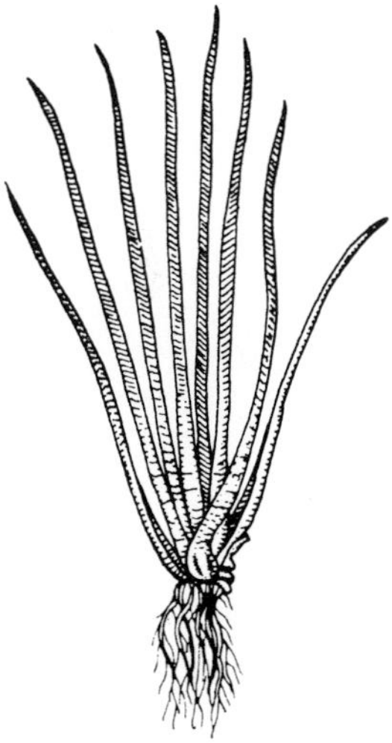

Isoetes muelleri

von MUELLER, Baron Ferdinand Jakob Heinrich (1825–1896)

Major contributions to medicine, exploration, scholarship and civic life –

Pharmacist, Botanist, Explorer,
Gardener, Patron of Science

Countries of residence and civic and scientific contribution –

Germany (Rostock, Kiel)
Australia (Adelaide, Melbourne)

Scientific Names –

Austromuellera trinervia (a monotypic genus)
Muellerina spp.
Boronia muelleri
Glochidion ferdinandii

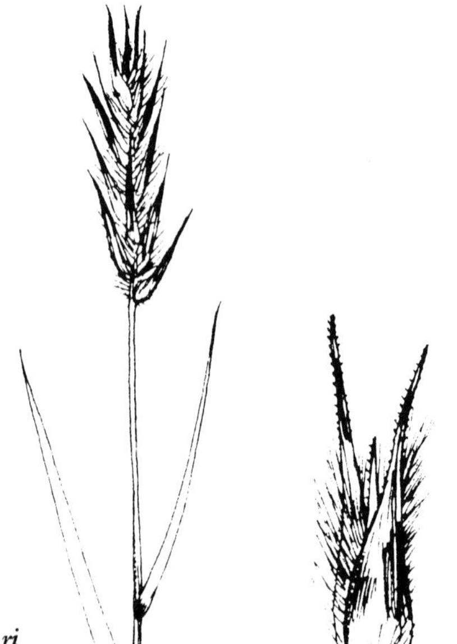

Paraneurachne muelleri

MURRAY, Surgeon James Patrick (*c.* 1839–*c.* 1885)

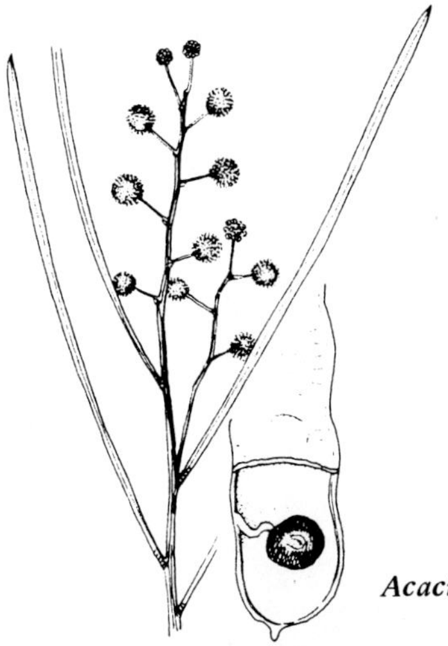

Acacia murrayana

Major contributions to medicine, exploration, scholarship and civic life –

Surgeon, Botanist, Writer,
Military Surgeon, Murderer

Countries of residence and civic and scientific contribution –

Ireland (Dublin), England (Manchester),
Australia (Melbourne, Queensland),
New Zealand (Invercargill),
South Pacific

Scientific Name – Acacia murrayana

MURRAY, Professor Johan Andreas (1740–1791)

Major contributions to medicine, exploration, scholarship and civic life –

Physician, Botanist, Professor of Medicine

Countries of residence and civic and scientific contribution –

Sweden (Stockholm), Germany (Göttingen)

Scientific Name – Murraya spp.

MUSA, Antonius (63 B.C. – 14 B.C.)

Major contributions to medicine, exploration, scholarship and civic life –

Physician, Writer

Country of residence and civic and scientific contribution –

Rome

Scientific Name – Musa spp.

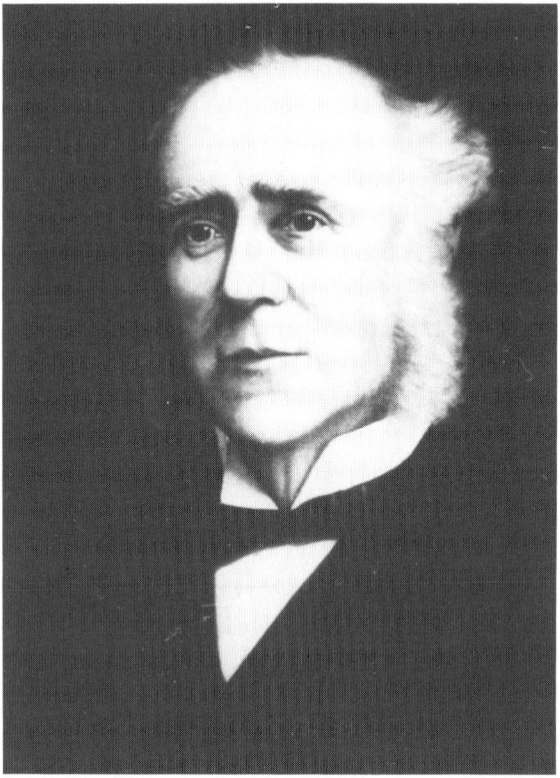

Dr JAMES EDWARD NEILD (1824–1906)

Physician and journalist, forensic pathologist and drama critic, of Melbourne.

Great patron of medicine, medical education and the arts, his name is commemorated in Darwinia neildiana, or Neild's Scent-Myrtle.

Photo, courtesy of the Victorian Branch of St John Ambulance Australia, of which he was a founder.

NEES von ESENBECK, Professor Theodor Friedrich Ludwig (1787–1837)

Major contributions to medicine, exploration, scholarship and civic life –

Pharmacist, Professor of Pharmacy, Botanist, Garden Inspector

Country of residence and civic and scientific contribution –

Germany (Odenwalde, Bonn)

Scientific Name – Drosera neesii

NEILD, Dr James Edward (1824–1906)

Major contributions to medicine, exploration, scholarship and civic life –

Physician, Journalist, Drama Critic, Forensic Specialist, Medical Editor, Goldminer, Patron of First Aid, University Lecturer, Orator

Countries of residence and civic and scientific contribution –

England (Yorkshire, Sheffield, Rochdale)
Australia (Castlemaine, Melbourne)

Scientific Name – Darwinia neildiana

NICANDER, (*fl.* 185 B.C. – 135 B.C.)

Major contributions to medicine, exploration, scholarship and civic life –

Physician, Botanist, Zoologist, Poet

Country of residence and civic and scientific contribution –

Greece (Colophon)

Scientific Name –

Nicandra spp. (an introduced weed, now naturalized)

NICHOLSON, Sir Charles (1808–1903)

Major contributions to medicine, exploration, scholarship and civic life –

Physician, Obstetrician, Pastoralist, Businessman, Parliamentarian, Collector, Philanthropist, Scholar, University Chancellor, Archaeologist

Countries of residence and civic and scientific contribution –

England (Cumberland, Yorkshire, London), Scotland (Edinburgh), Australia (Sydney, Port Phillip, Queensland), Egypt, Channel Islands, Denmark (Jutland)

Scientific Name – Goodenia nicholsonii

NEIMEYER, Professor Felix

Major contributions to medicine, exploration, scholarship and civic life –

Physician, Pathologist

Country of residence and civic and scientific contribution –

Germany (Tübingen)

Scientific Name – Niemeyera spp.

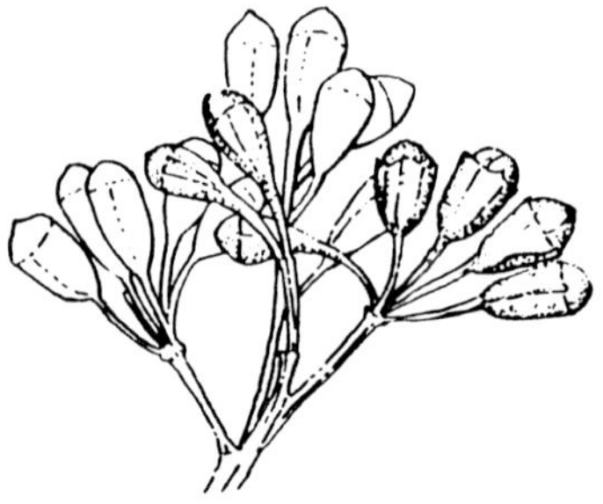

OSBORNE, Professor William (1873–1967)

Major contributions to medicine, exploration, scholarship and civic life –

Physiologist, Biochemist, Inventor, Writer, Dean of Medicine, Nutritionalist, Patron of Literature and Radio

Countries of residence and civic and scientific contribution –

Ireland (Belfast), Germany (Tübingen), England (London), Australia (Melbourne)

Scientific Name – Gilruthia osbornii

OTTAVIANI, Dr Vincent (eighteenth century)

Major contributions to medicine, exploration, scholarship and civic life –

Doctor, Botanist

Country of residence and civic and scientific contribution –

Italy

Scientific Name –

Octaviania spp. (e.g. *O. clelandi*, a large fungus of South Australia)

OWEN, Sir Richard (1804–1892)

Major contributions to medicine, exploration, scholarship and civic life –

Doctor, Anatomist, Palaeontologist, Museum Curator

Country of residence and civic and scientific contribution –

England (Lancashire, London)

Scientific Name – Owenia spp.

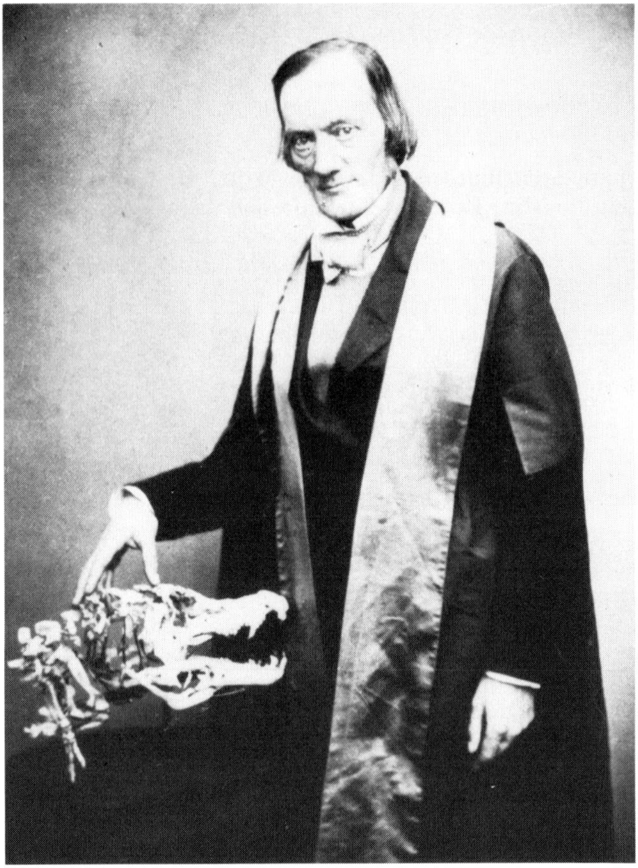

SIR RICHARD OWEN (1804–1892)

Doctor and anatomist, and first Hunterian Professor of Comparative Anatomy and Physiology at the Royal College of Surgeons in London.

His first paper to The Royal Society was on the mammary gland of the platypus. He was the foundation Curator of the British Museum of Natural History and is commemorated in the six species of the genus Owenia, found only in Australia. One – O. acidula, is called the Emu Apple tree.

Photograph courtesy of The National Portrait Gallery, London.

PAGET, Sir James (1814–1899)

Major contributions to medicine, exploration, scholarship and civic life –

Surgeon, Anatomist, Botanist, Historian

Country of residence and civic and scientific contribution –

England (Yarmouth, Cambridge, London)

Scientific Name – *Pagetia* spp.

PALMER, Sir James Frederick (1803–1871)

Major contributions to medicine, exploration, scholarship and civic life –

Surgeon, Army Surgeon, Anatomist, Businessman, Pastoralist, Churchman, Parliamentarian, Educationalist, Mayor of Melbourne

Countries of residence and civic and scientific contribution –

England (Devon, London), Australia (Melbourne)

Scientific Name – *Palmeria* spp.

PARKINSON, John (1567–1650)

Major contributions to medicine, exploration, scholarship and civic life –

Apothecary, Botanist, Herbalist, Gardener

Country of residence and civic and scientific contribution –

England (Nottingham, London)

Scientific Name –

Parkinsonia spp. (an introduced genus, now naturalized)

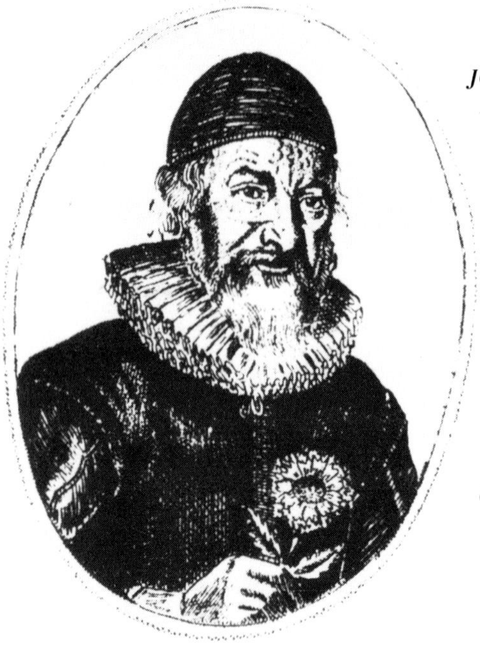

JOHN PARKINSON (1560–1650) Apothecary and Kings's Herbalist, of London. He established a "Physicale Garden of Simples" at Long Acre in a Parish of St Martin-in-the-Fields in what is now central London. His love of flowers and herbs and his gardening skills transformed the garden into a "Theater of Plantes".

Engraving courtesy of the "Cottage Gardener and Country Gentleman", 1875.

PARLATORE, Professor Filippo (1816–1877)

Major contributions to medicine, exploration, scholarship and civic life –

Pharmacist, Botanist, Professor of Anatomy (Palermo),
Professor of Botany (Florence)

Country of residence and civic and scientific contribution –

Italy (Sicily, Florence)

Scientific Name – Callitris parlatorei

PARSONS, Dr James (1705–1770)

Major contributions to medicine, exploration, scholarship and civic life –

Physician, Natural Historian, Anatomist,
Collector & Antiquary, Scholar, Linguist

Countries of residence and civic and scientific contribution –

England (Devon, London), Ireland, France

Scientific Name – Parsonsia spp.

PASCAL, Professor Didaco Baldassare (1768–1812)

Major contributions to medicine, exploration, scholarship and civic life –

Physician

Country of residence and civic and scientific contribution –

Italy (Parma)

Scientific Name – Pascalia spp. (syn. *Wedelia*)

Cephaelis ipecacuanha, a Brazilian ipecac, from the notebook of the surgeon-botanist WILLIAM PISO (1596–1648). Ipecac, containing the substance emetine, is used extensively to induce vomiting in children who have swallowed harmful tablets and poisons. The Australian tree, Pisonia, common on islands of the Great Barrier Reef, commemorates Piso's pioneering work in medical botany.

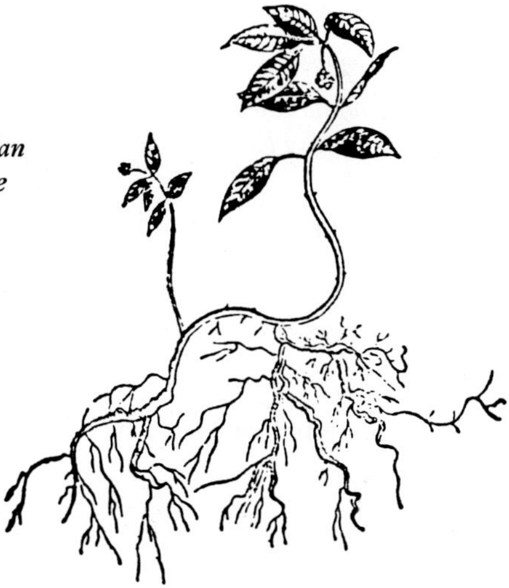

PISO, Dr Willem (1596–1648)

Major contributions to medicine, exploration, scholarship and civic life –

Doctor, Botanist, Explorer, Pharmacist

Countries of residence and civic and scientific contribution –

Holland (Leiden, Amsterdam), Brazil, Germany

Scientific Name – Pisonia spp.

PLANCHON, Professor Jules-Émile (1823–1888)

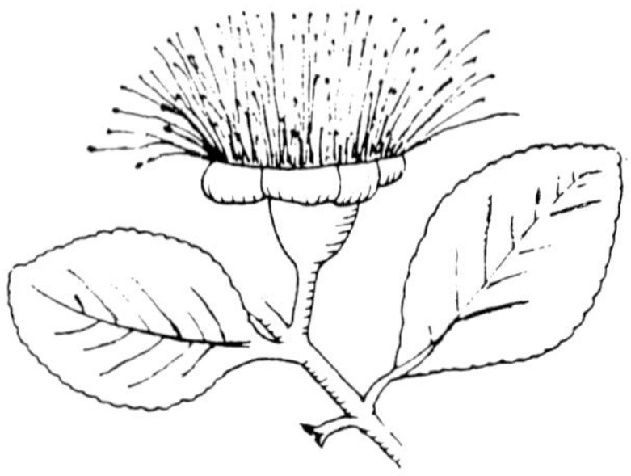

Planchonia careya

Major contributions to medicine, exploration, scholarship and civic life –

Physician, Botanist,
Plant Pathologist,
Professor of Medicine,
Agronomist

Countries of residence and civic and scientific contribution –

France (Montpellier, Nancy),
Belgium (Ghent), England (London),
United States of America

Scientific Names –

Planchonia careya (a sole species in Australia)
Eucalyptus planchoniana

PLANCHON, Professor Louis David (1858–1915)

Major contributions to medicine, exploration, scholarship and civic life –

Physician, Botanist, Pharmacologist, Professor of Materia Medica

Country of residence and civic and scientific contribution –

France (Montpellier, Paris)

Scientific Names –

Planchonella spp.
Drosera planchonii

PRENTICE, Dr Charles Brightly (1820–1894)

Major contributions to medicine, exploration, scholarship and civic life –

Surgeon, Botanist, Zoologist

Countries of residence and civic and scientific contribution –

England (Suffolk, Exeter), Australia (Brisbane)

Scientific Name – Panicum prenticeanum

PRINGLE, Sir John (1707–1782)

Major contributions to medicine, exploration, scholarship and civic life –

Physician, Military Physician, Preventive Medicine Exponent, Humanitarian

Countries of residence and civic and scientific contribution –

England (Roxburgh, London), Scotland (Edinburgh), Holland (Leiden), Europe

Scientific Name – Pringlea antiscorbutica

PULTENEY, Surgeon Richard (1730–1801)

Major contributions to medicine, exploration, scholarship and civic life –

Surgeon, Physician, Botanist, Historian

Country of residence and civic and scientific contribution –

England (Leicester, Loughborough, Blandford)

Scientific Name – Pultenaea spp.

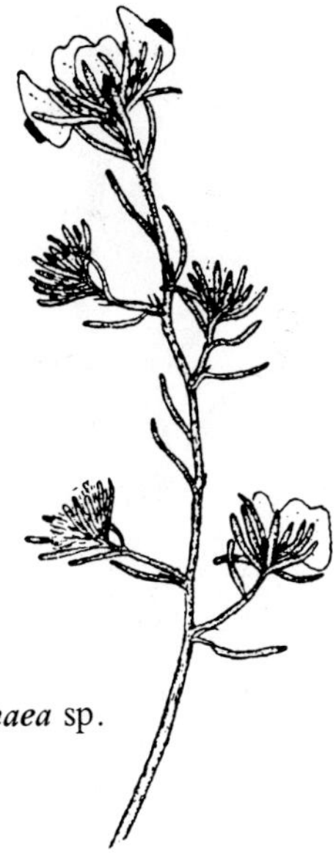

Pultenaea sp.

QUOY, Surgeon Jean Rene Constant (1790–1869)

Major contributions to medicine, exploration, scholarship and civic life –

Surgeon, Naval Surgeon, Naturalist

Countries of residence, and civic and scientific contribution –

France
Australia (Western Australia, Port Jackson, Tasmania)

Scientific Name –

Quoya spp. (syn. *Pityrodia*)

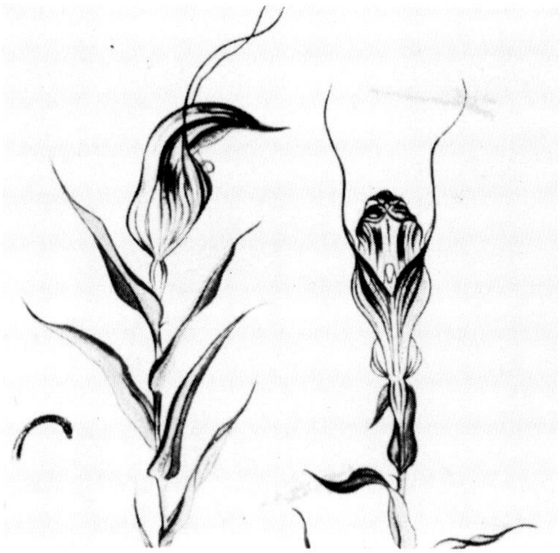

***Pterostylis rogersii*, a greenhood orchid named to commemorate the Adelaide physician and botanist, Dr RICHARD SANDERS ROGERS (1862–1942).**

RAND, Isaac (*c.* 1680–1743)

Major contributions to medicine, exploration, scholarship and civic life –

Apothecary, Gardener, Botanist

Country of residence and civic and scientific contribution –

England (London)

Scientific Name – Randia spp.

RICHE, Surgeon Claude Antoine Gaspar (1762–1797)

Major contributions to medicine, exploration, scholarship and civic life –

Surgeon, Naval Surgeon, Botanist, Collector

Countries of residence and civic and scientific contribution –

France (Montpellier), Australia (Western Australia)

Scientific Name – Richea spp.

ROBERTSON, Dr Barbara (born 1957)

Major contributions to medicine, exploration, scholarship and civic life –

Anaesthetist

Country of residence and civic and scientific contribution –

Australia (Melbourne)

Scientific Name –

Dahlia bipinnata "Barbara Robertson"

RODWAY, Dr Frederick Arthur (1880–1956)

Major contributions to medicine, exploration, scholarship and civic life –

Doctor, Botanist, Zoologist, Collector

Country of residence, and civic and scientific contribution –

Australia (Western Australia, Nowra)

Scientific Name – Aizoon rodwayi

ROGERS, Dr Richard Sanders (1862–1942)

Major contributions to medicine, exploration, scholarship and civic life –

Physician, Psychiatrist, Forensic Pathologist, Military Doctor, Botanist

Country of residence and civic and scientific contribution –

Australia (Adelaide)

Scientific Name – Pterostylis rogersii

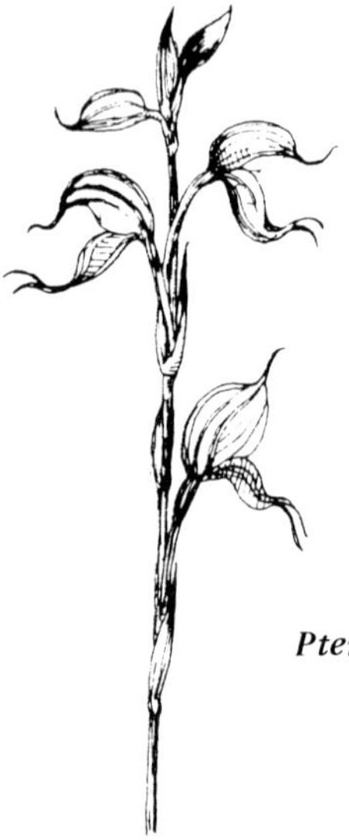

Pterostylis sp.

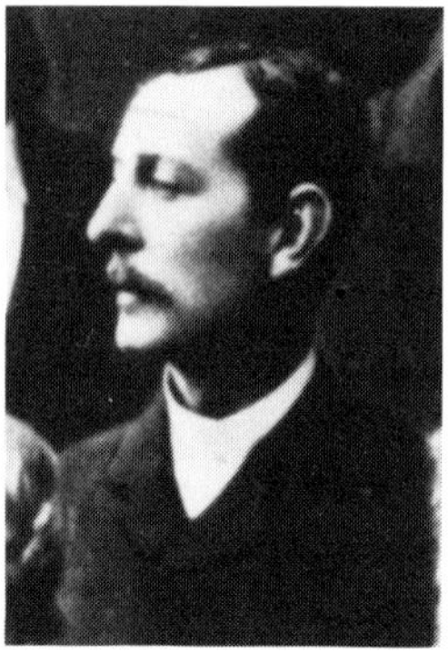

Dr WALTER EDMUND ROTH (1861–1933) Doctor, anthropologist and explorer, of Queensland. The native pepper of the North Queensland rainforests, Piper rothianum commemorates him.

ROTH, Dr Walter Edmund (1861–1933)

Major contributions to medicine, exploration, scholarship and civic life –

Doctor, Anthropologist, Explorer, Botanist, Teacher,
Magistrate, District Commissioner, Collector, Linguist

Countries of residence and civic and scientific contribution –

England (Oxford, London), Australia (Brisbane, Normanton,
Cloncurry, Cooktown), Guyana (Georgetown)

Scientific Names –

Piper rothianum
Anthurus rothae (a fungus)

ROTTBOELL, Professor Christen Friis (1727–1797)

Major contributions to medicine, exploration, scholarship and civic life –

Physician, Botanist, Gardener, Professor of Medicine

Countries of residence and civic and scientific contribution –

Denmark (Copenhagen), Sweden, France

Scientific Name – Rottboellia spp.

ROXBURGH, Dr William (1751–1815)

Major contributions to medicine, exploration, scholarship and civic life –

Doctor, Navy Surgeon, Botanist, Scientist, Gardener

Countries of residence and civic and scientific contribution –

Scotland (Ayrshire, Edinburgh), South Africa (Cape of Good Hope),
England (London), St Helena, India (Madras, Calcutta)

Scientific Name – Rotala roxburghiana

RUDALL, Dr James Thomas (1828–1907)

Major contributions to medicine, exploration, scholarship and civic life –
Surgeon, Naval Surgeon, Ophthalmologist, ENT Surgeon, Musician

Countries of residence, and civic and scientific contribution –
England (London), Arctic, Australia (Melbourne)

Scientific Name – Myriocephalus rudallii

du RUEL, Jean (1479–1537)

Major contributions to medicine, exploration, scholarship and civic life –
Physician, Herbalist, Canon, Translator, "Dean" of Medicine

Country of residence and civic and scientific contribution –
France (Paris)

Scientific Name – Ruellia spp. (syn. *Brunoniella*)

RUELING, Dr Johann Philipp (1741–1803)

Major contributions to medicine, exploration, scholarship and civic life –
Physician, Botanist, Zoologist

Country of residence and civic and scientific contribution –
Germany (Göttingen, Einbeck, Nordheim)

Scientific Name – Rulingia spp.

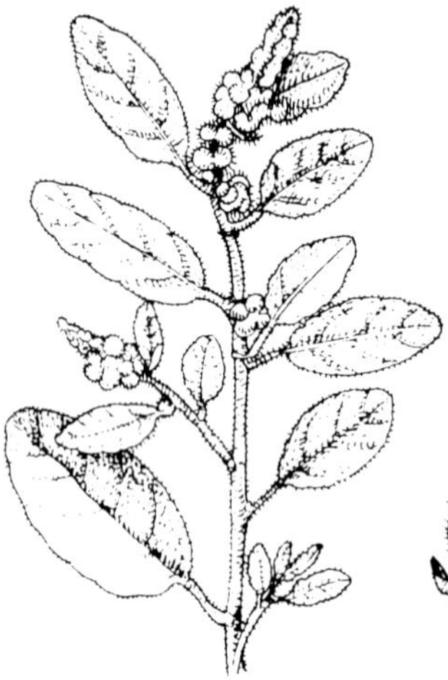

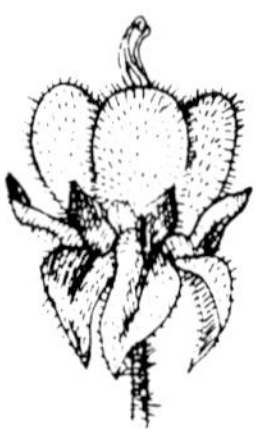

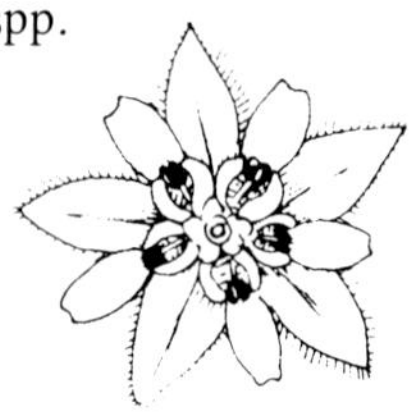

Rulingia loxophylla

SCHELHAMMER, Professor Gustav Christoph (1649–1716)

Major contributions to medicine, exploration, scholarship and civic life –

Physician, Professor of Anatomy, Surgery and Botany

Country of residence and civic and scientific contribution –

Germany (Helmstadt, Gena, Kiel)

Scientific Name – Schelhammera spp.

SCHOEN, Johannes Matthias Albrecht (early 19th century)

Major contributions to medicine, exploration, scholarship and civic life –

Ophthalmologist

Country of residence and civic and scientific contribution –

Germany (Hamburg)

Scientific Name – Schoenia cassiniana (a monotypic genus)

SCHOLTZ, Dr Johann Eduard Heinrich (1812–1859)

Major contributions to medicine, exploration, scholarship and civic life –

Doctor, Botanist, Zoologist

Country of residence and civic and scientific contribution –

Germany (Breslau, Göttingen)

Scientific Name – Scholtzia spp.

SHUTER, Dr James (? –1834)

Major contributions to medicine, exploration, scholarship and civic life –

Doctor, Botanist, Naturalist

Countries of residence, and civic and scientific contribution –

India (Madras), England

Scientific Name –

Shuteria vestita (one species only in Australia)

SIEGESBECK, Dr Johann Georg (1686–1755)

Major contributions to medicine, exploration, scholarship and civic life –

Apothecary, Gardener, Botanist

Country of residence and civic and scientific contribution –

Russia (Leningrad, Seehausen, Helmstedt)

Scientific Name –

Sigesbeckia orientalis (one species only in Australia)

SLOANE, Sir Hans (1660–1753)

Major contributions to medicine, exploration, scholarship and civic life –

Physician, Scholar, Scientist, Natural Historian,
Military Physician, Museum Curator

Countries of residence and civic and scientific contribution –

Ireland (County Down), France (Paris, Montpellier),
England (London), Jamaica

Scientific Name – Sloanea spp.

SMITH, Sir James Edward (1759–1828)

Major contributions to medicine, exploration, scholarship and civic life –

Physician, Philanthropist, Botanist

Countries of residence and civic and scientific contribution –

England (Norwich, London), Scotland (Edinburgh),
Holland (Leiden)

Scientific Name – Smithia spp.

SOLANDER, Dr Daniel Carol (1733–1782)

Major contributions to medicine, exploration, scholarship and civic life –

Botanist, Natural Historian, Doctor, Cataloguer, Librarian

Countries of residence and civic and scientific contribution –

Sweden (Uppsala), England (London, Oxford),
Australia, South Pacific, Iceland

Scientific Name – Acacia solandri

SOLLY, Dr Richard Horsman (1778–1858)

Major contributions to medicine, exploration, scholarship and civic life –

Physiologist, Anatomist

Country of residence and civic and scientific contribution –

England (London)

Scientific Name – Sollya spp.

STEETZ, Joachim (1804–1862)

Major contributions to medicine, exploration, scholarship and civic life –
Pharmacist, Doctor, Botanist, Zoologist

Country of residence and civic and scientific contribution –
Germany (Halle, Wurzburg, Hamburg)

Scientific Name – Waitzia steetziana

STEPHENSON, Surgeon William (*c.* 1792–1863)

Major contributions to medicine, exploration, scholarship and civic life –
Surgeon, Military Surgeon, Naturalist, Explorer, Collector

Countries of residence and civic and scientific contribution –
India, China, Australia (Northern Territory, Queensland, Taree)

Scientific Name –

Platysace stephensonii
(formerly *Trachymene stephensonii,*
formerly *Siebera stephensonii*)

SURIAN, Dr Joseph Donat (? –1691)

Major contributions to medicine, exploration, scholarship and civic life –
Doctor, Analytical Chemist

Countries of residence and civic and scientific contribution –
France (Marseilles), Antilles

Scientific Name –
Suriana maritima (a monotypic genus)

SUTTON, Dr Charles Stanford (*c.* 1865–1950)

Major contributions to medicine, exploration, scholarship and civic life –
Doctor, Botanist, Collector

Country of residence and civic and scientific contribution –
Australia (Victoria, especially Melbourne)

Scientific Names –
Prasophyllum suttonii
Pterostylis suttonii

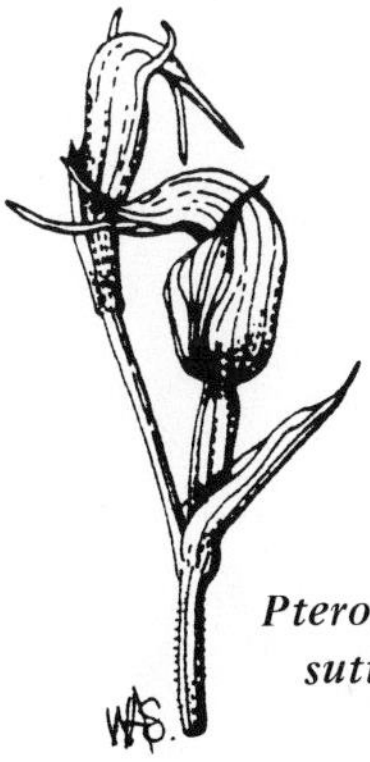

Pterostylis suttonii

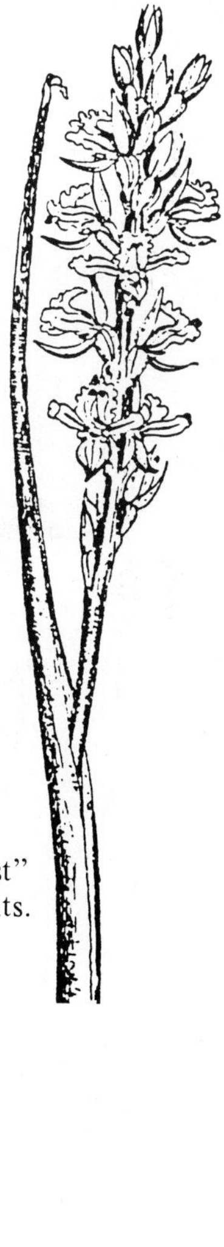

Prasophyllum suttonii
Courtesy of "Victorian Naturalist" 1933, with acknowledgements.

Medicine and Botany

SWAINSON, Dr Isaac (1746–1812)

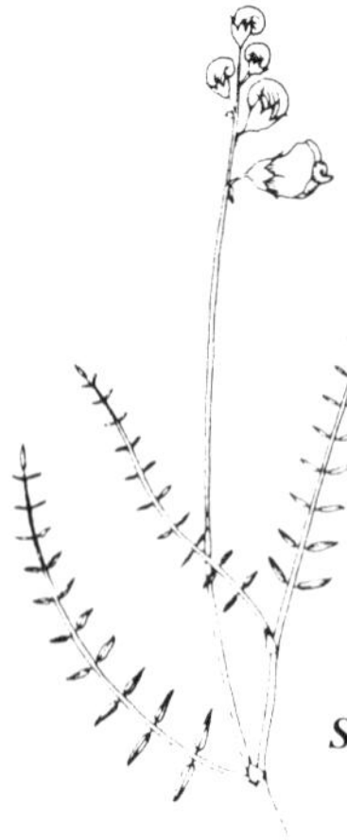

Swainsona procumbens

Major contributions to medicine, exploration, scholarship and civic life –

Doctor, Botanist, Gardener

Countries of residence and civic and scientific contribution –

England (London), Australia

Scientific Name – Swainsona spp.

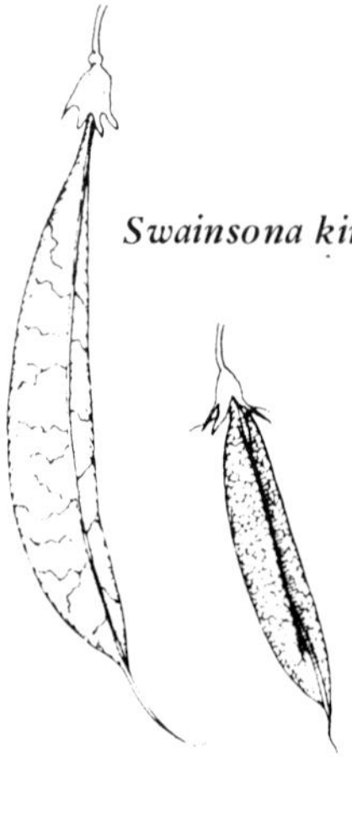

Swainsona kingii

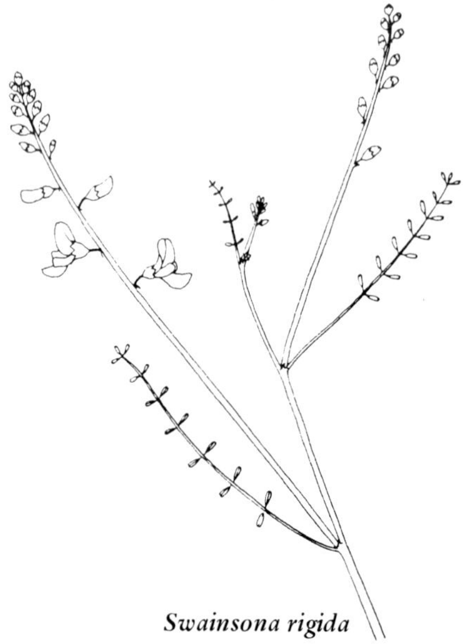

Swainsona rigida

TATE, Dr Thomas (1842–1934)

Major contributions to medicine, exploration, scholarship and civic life –

Medical Student, Doctor, Ship's Surgeon, Explorer, Botanist, Collector

Countries of residence and civic and scientific contribution –

England (Northumberland), Australia (Cape York, Brisbane, Rockhampton)

Scientific Name – Premna tateana

TEUCER, King of Troy (*c.* 1400–*c.* 1000 B.C.)

Major contributions to medicine, exploration, scholarship and civic life –

First King of Troy, Healer

Country of residence and civic and scientific contribution –

Troy (now in Asia Minor as part of Turkey)

Scientific Name – Teucrium spp.

THEOPHRASTOS, Eresios (*c.*372 B.C.–*c.* 287 B.C.)

Major contributions to medicine, exploration, scholarship and civic life –

Philosopher, Doctor, Natural Historian, Teacher, Ethicist

Country of residence and civic and scientific contribution –

Greece (Lesbos, Macedonia, Athens)

Scientific Name – Abutilon theophrasti

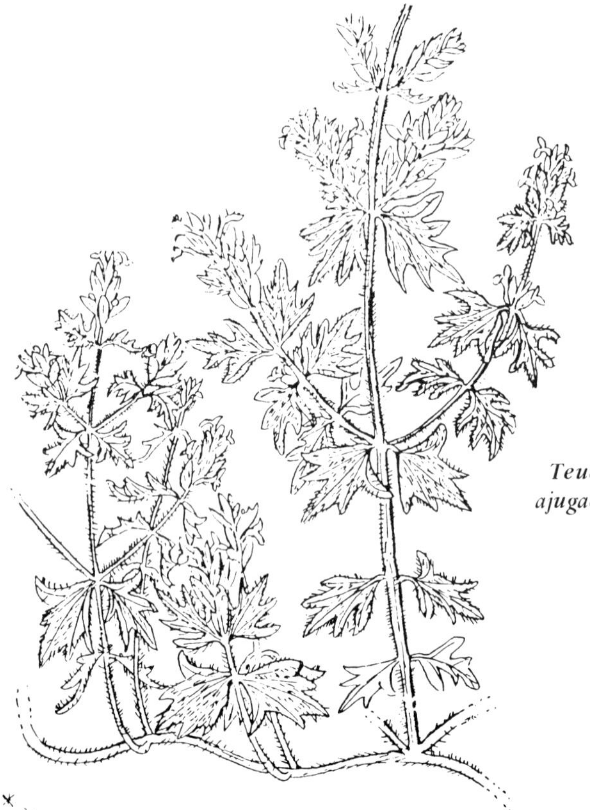

Teucrium ajugaceum

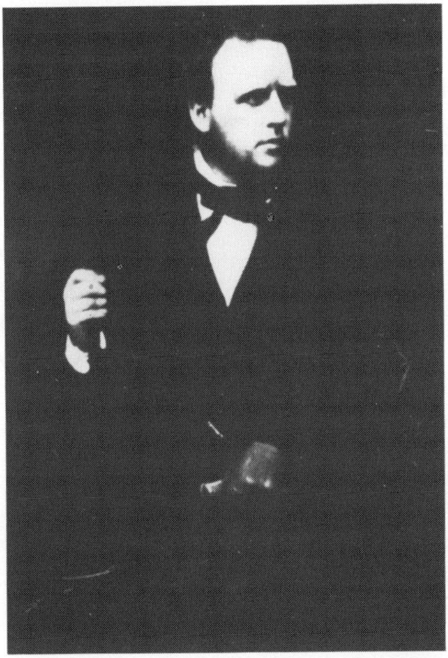

Dr DAVID JOHN THOMAS (1813–1871)

Pioneering Melbourne surgeon. The West Australian plant Chamaelaucium thomasii (Thomas's Wax-plant) bears his name.

Photo courtesy of the Australian Medical Association (Victorian Branch), and Mr Ron Hastings.

THOMAS, Dr David John (1813–1871)

Major contributions to medicine, exploration, scholarship and civic life –

Surgeon, Apothecary, Ship's Surgeon, Anatomist,
Psychiatrist, Humanist

Countries of residence and civic and scientific contribution –

Wales (Llangadock, Swansea), England (London),
Australia (Tasmania, Melbourne)

Scientific Name – Chamaelaucium thomasii

THRELKELD, Dr Caleb ((1676–1728)

Major contributions to medicine, exploration, scholarship and civic life –

Physician, Churchman, Botanist, Gardener

Countries of residence and civic and scientific contribution –

England (Cumberland),
Scotland (Glasgow, Edinburgh),
Ireland (Dublin)

Scientific Name – *Threlkeldia* spp.

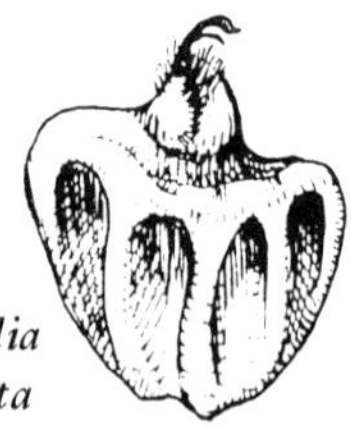

Threlkeldia incboata

THUNBERG, Professor Carl Peter (1743–1828)

Major contributions to medicine, exploration, scholarship and civic life –

Botanist, Physician, Teacher

Countries of residence and civic and scientific contribution –

Sweden (Uppsala), South Africa (Cape of Good Hope),
Japan (Nagasaki), Java

Scientific Name – *Thunbergia* spp.

de TOURNEFORT, Professor Joseph Pitton (1656–1708)

Major contributions to medicine, exploration, scholarship and civic life –

Botanist, Doctor

Countries of residence and civic and scientific contribution –

France (Montpellier, Aix, Paris), Spain, Eastern Mediterranean

Scientific Names –

Tournefortia spp. (syn. *Argusia* syn. *Messerschmidia*)
Brassica tourneforti (an introduced weed, now naturalized)

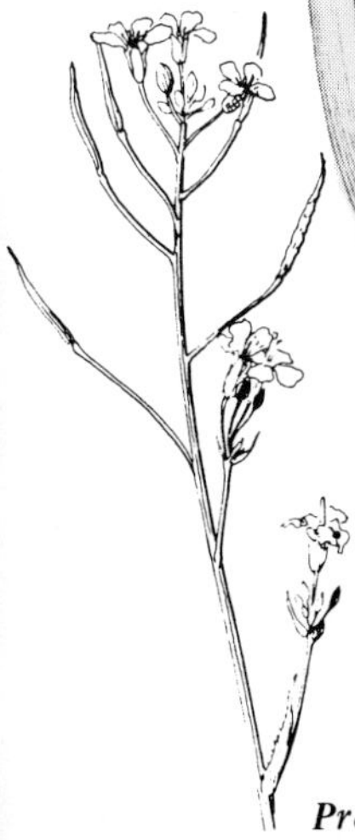

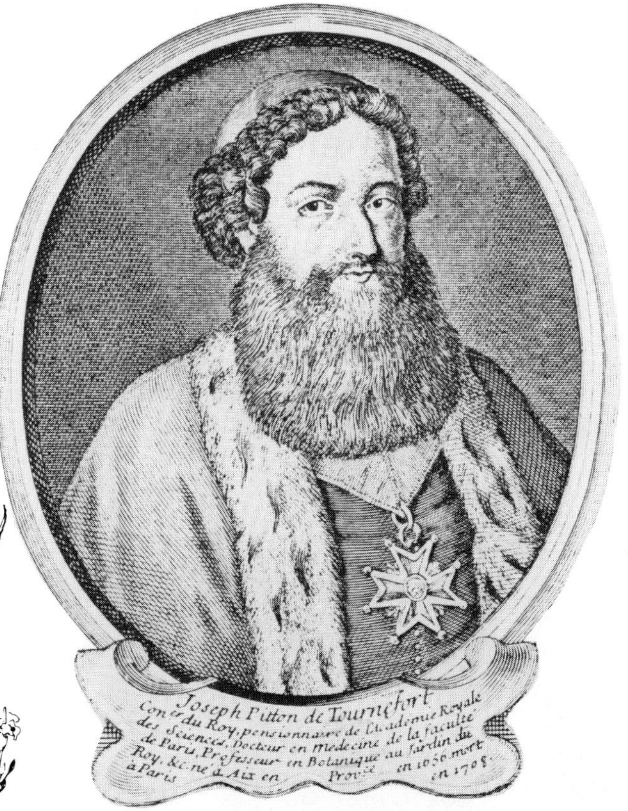

PROFESSOR JOSEPH PITTON de TOURNEFORT
(1656 – 1708)

Professor of Botany and (from 1706) Professor of Medicine at Paris. In 1698 he wrote "Histoire des plantes", with its full title "A History of Plants growing about Paris, with their uses in physick ..." In 1700 he published his herbal "Institutiones rei herbariae" which is one of the great books not only in the history of botany, but of science. He was one of the earliest taxonomists, introduced the concept of genera, and laid the foundations for much of Linnaeus' work. Two species of the genus Tournefortia are native to Australia, and the introduced weed Brassica tournefortia is widespread in the dry hot interior of Australia.

(Photo of a zinc engraving by J. Cederquist, with acknowledgements to Acta Horti Bergiani, Stockholm)

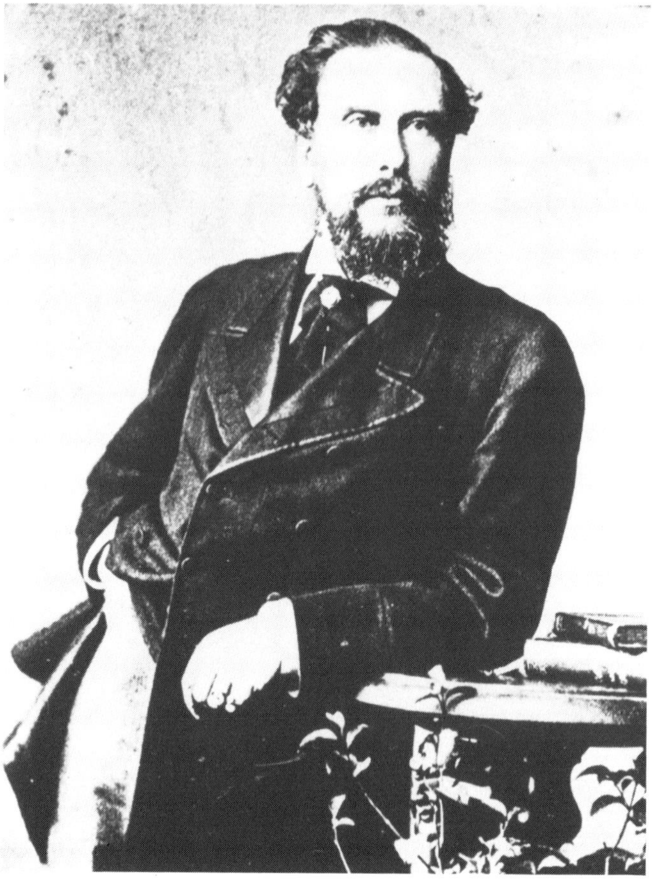

Dr RICHARD THOMAS TRACY
(1826 – 1874)

A founder of the Melbourne Lying-In Hospital and Infirmary for Diseases of Women and Children, later the Royal Women's Hospital, Melbourne.

Former goldminer, magistrate and churchman, his name is commemorated in the plant Premna tracyana, and in the Queensland tree Clerodendrum tracyanum.

Photo courtesy of The Royal Women's Hospital, Melbourne, and Ms Pamela McLure.

TRACY, Dr Richard Thomas (1826–1874)

Major contributions to medicine, exploration, scholarship and civic life –

Surgeon, Goldminer, Obstetrician, Paediatrician, Military Surgeon, University Lecturer, Physician, Churchman, Magistrate

Countries of residence and civic and scientific contribution –

Ireland (County Limerick, Dublin), England,
Australia (Adelaide, Bendigo, Melbourne)

Scientific Name – Premna tracyana

TRAGUS, Dr Jerome [syn. Dr Hieronymus Bock] (1498–1553)

Major contributions to medicine, exploration, scholarship and civic life –

School Teacher, Gardener, Preacher, Doctor

Country of residence and civic and scientific contribution –

Germany (Odenwald, Hornbach)

Scientific Names –

Tragus australianus (a grass)
Tragia novae-hollandiae (only one species in Australia)

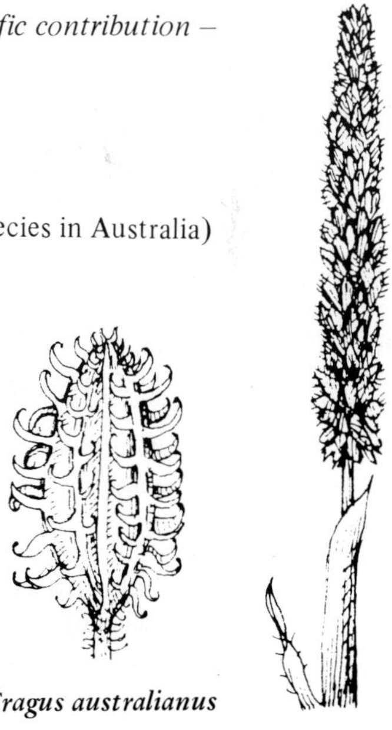

Tragus australianus

Tragia novae-hollandiae is not, as its literal translation suggests, an Australian goat, rather it is the sole Australian species of a widely distributed genus which commemorates Dr Hieronymus Tragus (1498–1553). Born Hieronymous Bock ("Tragos" is Greek for a billy-goat, "Bock" is the German term), he lived at Hornbach in Germany, being successively a schoolmaster, a curator of a great German garden, a preacher and then a physician.

(Photo courtesy of Acta Horti Bergiani, Stockholm)

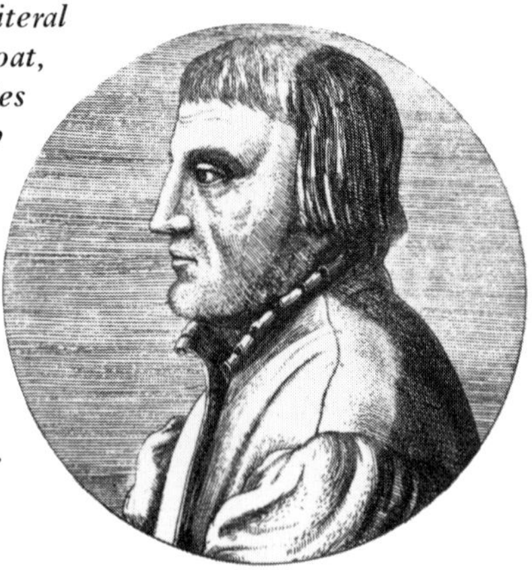

TRATMAN, Dr Frank (1860–1926)

Major contributions to medicine, exploration, scholarship and civic life –

Surgeon, Physician, Medical Officer of Health, Naturalist

Countries of residence and civic and scientific contribution –

England (Bristol, Guilford, London), Australia (Perth)

Scientific Name – Rulingia tratmanii

TRYON, Henry (1856–1943)

Major contributions to medicine, exploration, scholarship and civic life –

Medical Student, Naturalist, Scientist, Entomologist, Botanist, Toxinologist

Countries of residence and civic and scientific contribution –

England (Buckfastleigh), Sweden, New Zealand, Australia (Brisbane), New Guinea

Scientific Name – Bryum tryonii

VALLISNERI, Professor Antonio (1661–1730)

Major contributions to medicine, exploration, scholarship and civic life –

Physician, Naturalist, University Professor

Country of residence and civic and scientific contribution –

Italy (Bologna, Reggio, Padua)

Scientific Name – Vallisneria spp.

VILLARS, Professor Dominique (1745–1814)

Major contribution to medicine, exploration, scholarship and civic life –

Doctor, Botanist, Taxonomist

Country of residence and civic and scientific contribution –

France (Grenoble, Paris, Strasbourg)

Scientific Name – Villarsia spp.

VIRCHOW, Professor Rudolf (1821–1902)

Major contributions to medicine, exploration, scholarship and civic life –

Pathologist, Scientist, Military Doctor, Publisher,
Anatomist, Politician, Anthropologist and Archaeologist
Public Health Expert, Teacher

Country of residence and civic and scientific contribution –

Germany (Silesia, Wurzburg, Berlin)

Scientific Name – Ceratopetalum virchowii

VITTADINI, Dr Carlo (1800–1865)

Major contributions to medicine, exploration, scholarship and civic life –
Physician, Botanist

Country of residence and civic and scientific contribution –
Italy (Pavia, Torino, Milan)

Scientific Name – *Vittadinia* spp.

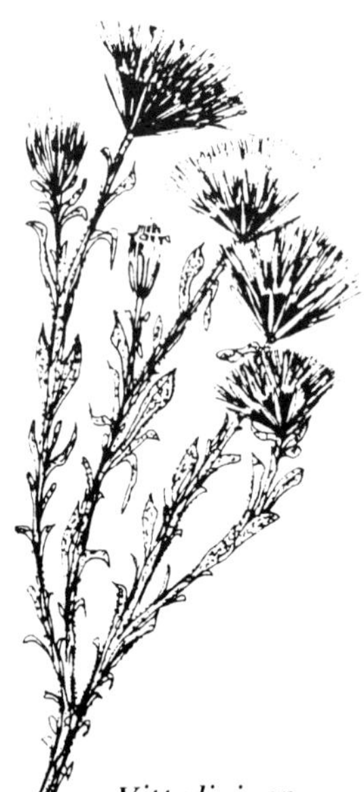

Vittadinia sp.

WAHLENBERG, Professor Goran (1780–1851)

Major contributions to medicine, exploration, scholarship and civic life –

Physician, Botanist, Taxonomist, Professor of Medicine

Countries of residence and civic and scientific contribution –

Sweden (Uppsala), Norway, Switzerland

Scientific Name – Wahlenbergia spp.

WAITZ, Dr Karl Friedrich (1774–1848)

Major contributions to medicine, exploration, scholarship and civic life –

Physician, Botanist, Collector

Countries of residence and civic and scientific contribution –

Germany (Altenburg, Bavaria), Indonesia (Semarang), Holland

Scientific Name – Waitzia spp.

WALTHER, Professor Augustin Friedrich (1688–1746)

Major contributions to medicine, exploration, scholarship and civic life –

Physician, Botanist

Country of residence and civic and scientific contribution –

Germany (Wittenburg, Leipzig)

Scientific Name – Waltheria spp.

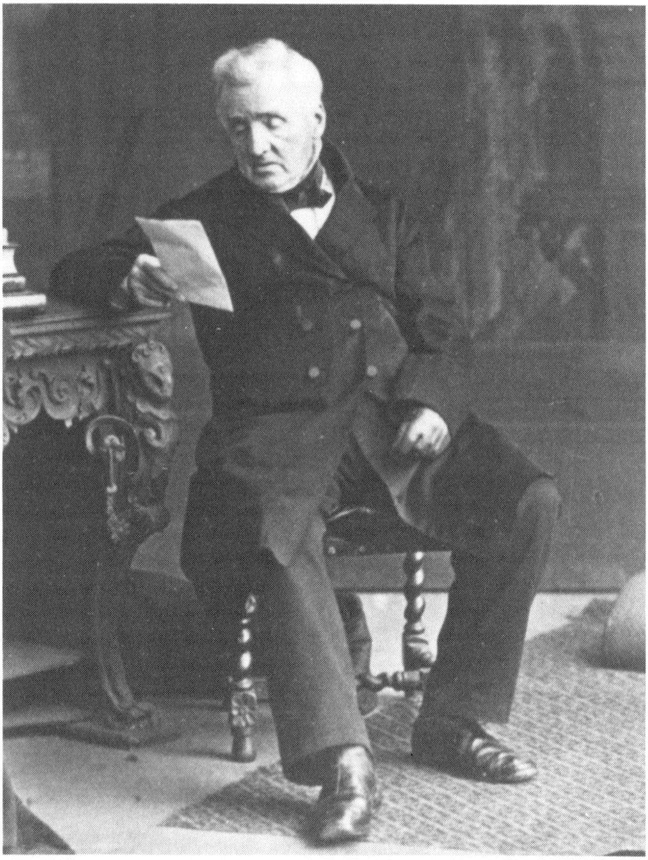

A contemplative Dr NATHANIEL BAGSHAW WARD (1791–1868)
An English physician and botanist, co-founder of the Microscopical Society and examiner to the Society of Apothecaries.

He invented an airtight glass container for transporting plants on long sea voyages. Now called the Wardian case, it allowed many Australian plants to reach the gardens of Europe alive. The glass allows light to penetrate, and the plants are watered by the nightly condensation of water which vaporizes during the day.
The popular indoor terrarium works on this principle.
Species of Amphiroa and Bostrychia also commemorate his name.

(Photo courtesy of The Hunt Institute for Botanical Documentation, Pittsburgh)

WARD, Dr Nathaniel Bagshaw (1791–1868)

Major contributions to medicine, exploration, scholarship and civic life –
Physician, Botanist, Inventor, Collector

Country of residence and civic and scientific contribution –
England (London)

Scientific Name – Amphiroa wardii

WATSON, Professor Archibald (1849–1940)

Major contributions to medicine, exploration, scholarship and civic life –
Anatomist, Explorer, Teacher, Professor of Anatomy

Countries of residence and civic and scientific contribution –
Australia (Adelaide, Wiluna), South Pacific

Scientific Name – Calytrix watsonii

WATSON, Sir William (1715–1787)

Major contributions to medicine, exploration, scholarship and civic life –
Physician, Paediatrician, Apothecary, Physicist, Botanist

Countries of residence and civic and scientific contribution –
England (London), Germany (Halle, Wittenburg)

Scientific Name –

Watsonia spp. (native to South Africa, six species are spread widely throughout southern Australia)

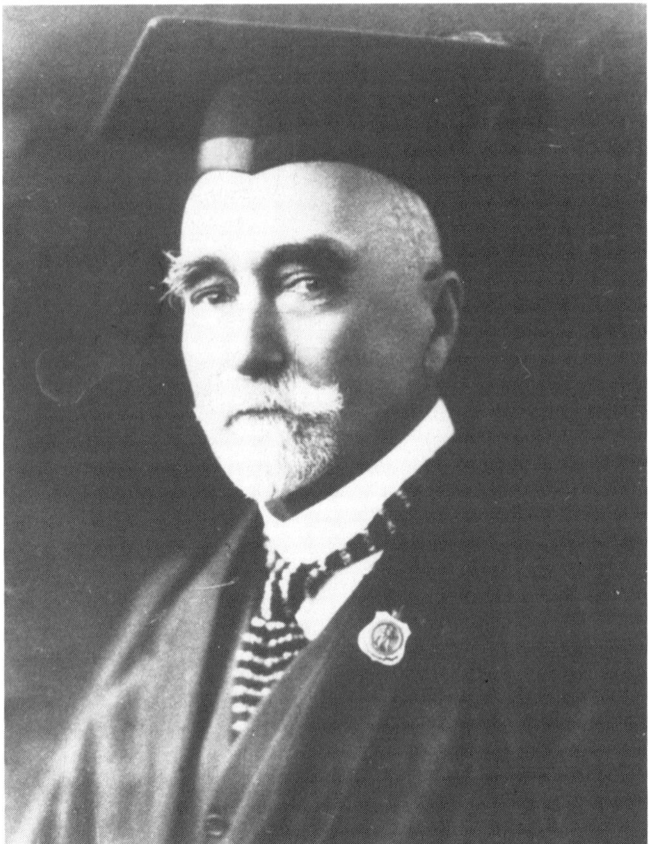

PROFESSOR ARCHIBALD WATSON
(1849 – 1940)

Anatomist, explorer and University teacher of Adelaide.
The two Australian plants Calytrix and Goodenia watsonii commemorate his life and works.

Photo courtesy the State Library of South Australia.

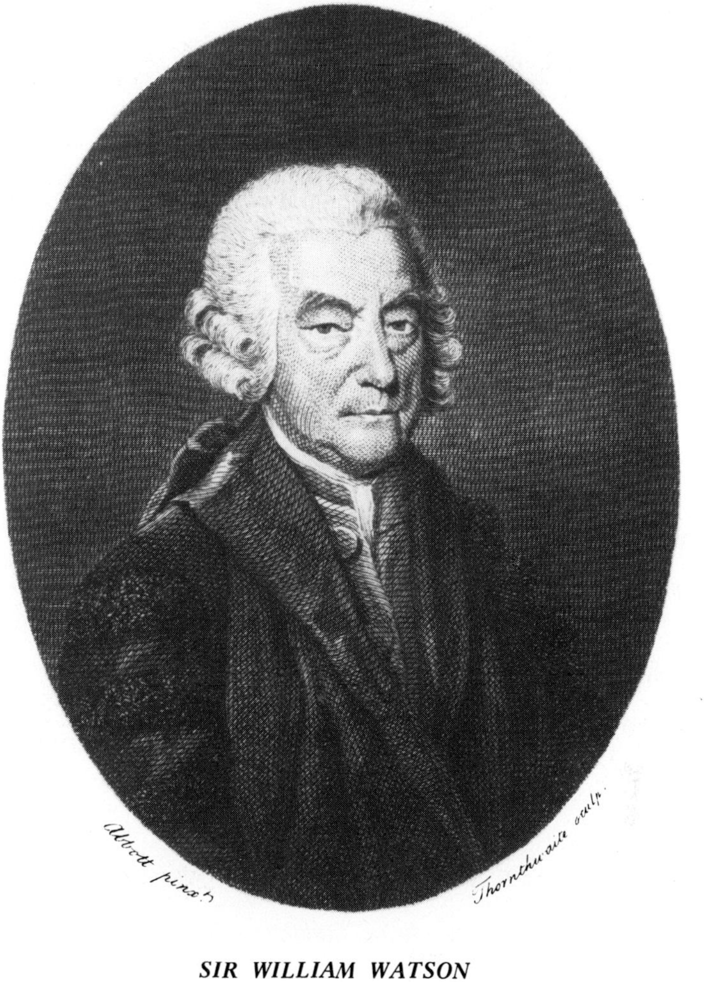

SIR WILLIAM WATSON
(1715 – 1789)

One of the world's first specialist paediatricians, and doctor to The Foundling Hospital, London.
Some six species of Watsonia, originally introduced from South Africa, occur widely in southern Australia.

Photo courtesy of the Royal Botanic Gardens, Kew, England, with acknowledgements.

WEBSTER, Dr Leonard Clarke (1870–1942)

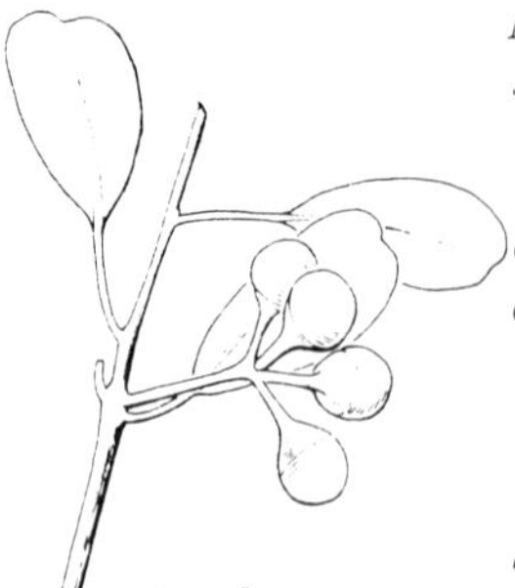

Eucalyptus websteriana

Major contributions to medicine, exploration, scholarship and civic life –

Doctor, Pharmacist, Botanist, Collector

Country of residence and civic and scientific contribution –

Australia (Coolgardie, Tasmania, New South Wales)

Scientific Name –

Eucalyptus websteriana

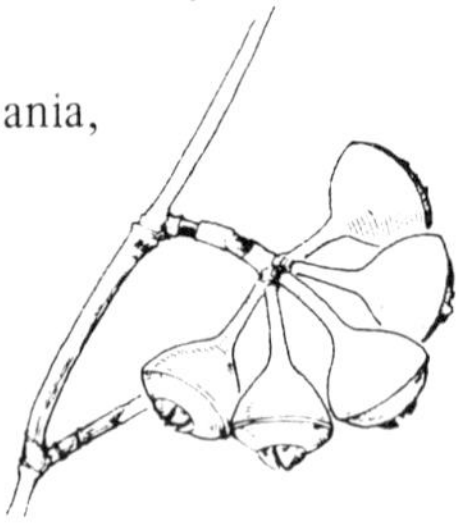

WEDEL, Professor George Wolfgang (1645–1721)

Major contributions to medicine, exploration, scholarship and civic life –

Physician, Botanist, Professor of Medicine

Country of residence and civic and scientific contribution –

Germany (Gotha, Jena)

Scientific Name – Wedelia spp.

WEHL, Dr Eduard (*c.* 1823–1876)

Major contributions to medicine, exploration, scholarship and civic life –

Physician

Countries of residence and civic and scientific contribution –

Germany, Australia (Guichen Bay, Mt Gambier)

Scientific Names –

Wehlia spp.
Gigartina wehliae

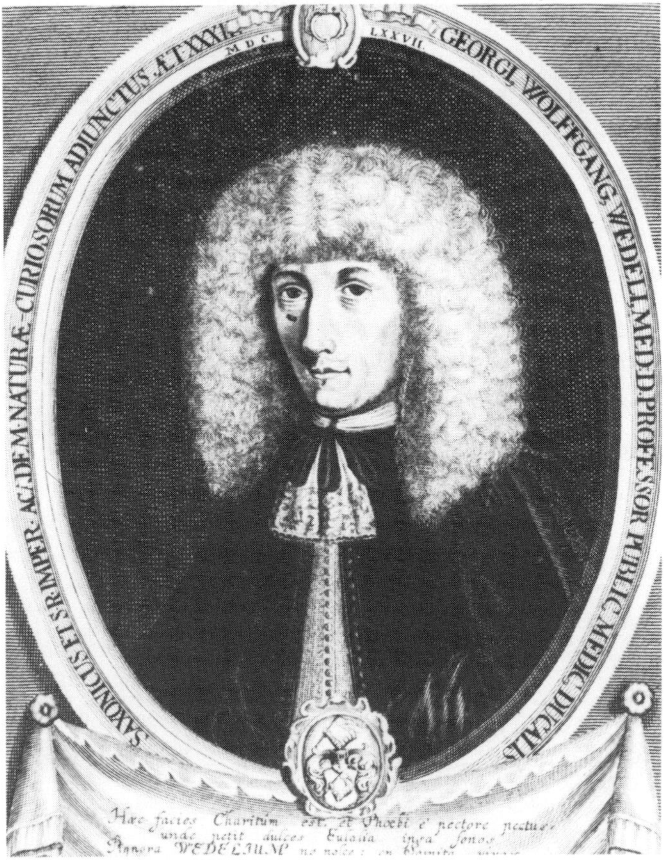

PROFESSOR GEORG WOLFGANG WEDEL
(1645 – 1721)
Professor of Medicine and botanist of Jena, now in East Germany.
There are six Australian species of plants in the genus Wedelia.
One of these, Wedelia asperrima ("yellow daisy") contains wedeloside
which is a potent toxin of mitochondria, the essential cellular
structures which are the site of respiration.
The familiar Wedia trilobata ("Singapore Daisy" or "Creeping Daisy")
is now grown extensively as ground cover in temperate and
northern Australia. It is an introduced species which also commemorates
(some would say too vigorously) this German doctor.

(Photo courtesy of The Hunt Institute for Botanical Documentation,
Carnegie-Mellon University, Pittsburgh.)

WEINMANN, Dr Johann Wilhelm (1683–1741)

Major contributions to medicine, exploration, scholarship and civic life –

Apothecary, Botanist

Country of residence and civic and scientific contribution –

Germany (Regensburg)

Scientific Name –

Weinmannia (Trans. *Ackama, Pseudoweinmannia*)

WESTRING, Dr Johan Petrus (1753–1833)

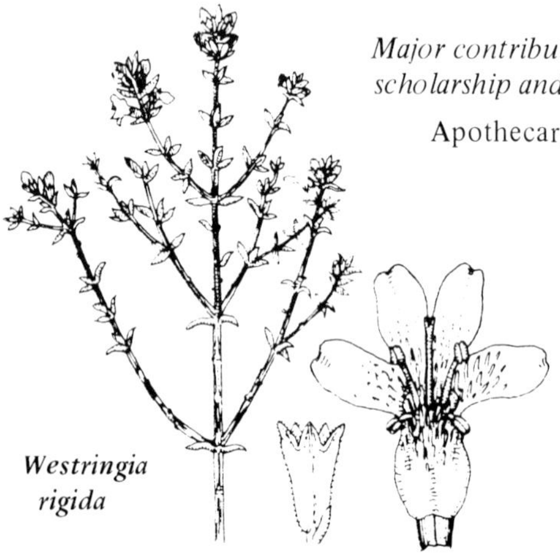

Westringia rigida

Major contributions to medicine, exploration, scholarship and civic life –

Apothecary, Botanist

Country of residence and civic and scientific contribution –

Sweden (Linkoping, Norrkoping, Uppsala)

Scientific Name –

Westringia spp.

WHEELER, Surgeon Walter Frank (*fl.* 1861)

Major contributions to medicine, exploration, scholarship and civic life –

Surgeon, Explorer, Botanist, Collector

Country of residence and civic and scientific contribution –

Australia (Victoria, Northern Territory)

Scientific Name – *Euphorbia wheeleri*

WILKIE, Dr David Elliot (1815–1885)

Major contributions to medicine, exploration, scholarship and civic life –

Physician, Surgeon, Obstetrician, Churchman,
Public Health Advocate, Patron of Arts, Inventor,
Parliamentarian

Countries of residence and civic and scientific contribution –

Scotland (Edinburgh), France (Paris),
Australia (Adelaide, Melbourne)

Scientific Name – Wilkiea spp.

WILLMOTT, Surgeon Julius John Eardley (1849–1897)

Major contributions to medicine, exploration, scholarship and civic life –

Surgeon, Paediatric Surgeon

Countries of residence and civic and scientific contribution –

Scotland (Aberdeen), Australia (Melbourne)

Scientific Name – Pentapanax willmottii (syn. *Polyscias willmottii*)

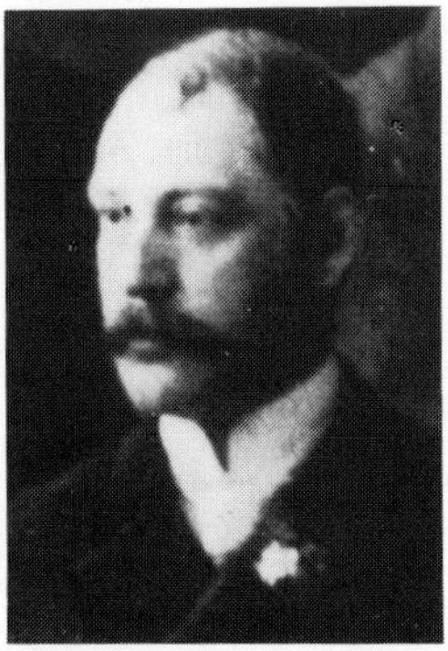

Dr Julius John Eardley Willmott, (1849–1897), a pioneering Australian paediatric surgeon, of Melbourne.

Photo, from the 1889 Intercolonial Medical Congress, Melbourne, courtesy of the Victorian Branch of the Australian Medical Association, and Mr Ron Hastings.

WILSON, Surgeon Thomas Braidwood (1792–1843)

Major contributions to medicine, exploration, scholarship and civic life –

Surgeon, Naval Surgeon, Surgeon-Superintendent of Convicts, Pastoralist

Countries of residence and civic and scientific contribution –

Scotland (West Lothian), East Indies,
Australia (Braidwood, Sydney, Tasmania)

Scientific Name – *Grevillea wilsoni*

von WOLFF, Dr Johann Friedrich (1778–1806)

Major contributions to medicine, exploration, scholarship and civic life –

Physician, Botanist

Country of residence and civic and scientific contribution –

Germany (Schweinfurt, Altorf)

Scientific Name – *Wolffia* spp.

WRIGHT, Physician-General William (1735–1819)

Major contributions to medicine, exploration, scholarship and civic life –

Physician, Naval Surgeon, Military Surgeon, Paediatrician, Botanist, Zoologist, Collector

Countries of residence and civic and scientific contribution –

Scotland (Crieff, Edinburgh), England (London), Greenland,
West Indies (Port Royal, St Pierre, Jamaica, Barbados)

Scientific Name – *Wrightia* spp.

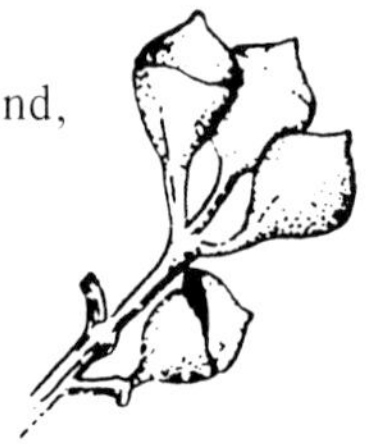

ZANNICHELLI, Dr Giovanni Girolamo (1662–1729)

Major contributions to medicine, exploration, scholarship and civic life –

Doctor, Pharmacist, Botanist

Country of residence and civic and scientific contribution –

Italy (Medena, Venice)

Scientific Name –

Zannichellia palustris
(Sole species, an aquatic plant, in Australia)

ZANTEDESCHI, Dr Giovanni (1773–1846)

Major contributions to medicine, exploration, scholarship and civic life –

Doctor, Botanist

Country of residence and civic and scientific contribution –

Italy (Verona, Padua)

Scientific Name –

Zantedeschia spp.
(a native of Africa; seen mostly in gardens where it is widely cultivated, but also seen in Australia as garden escapes)

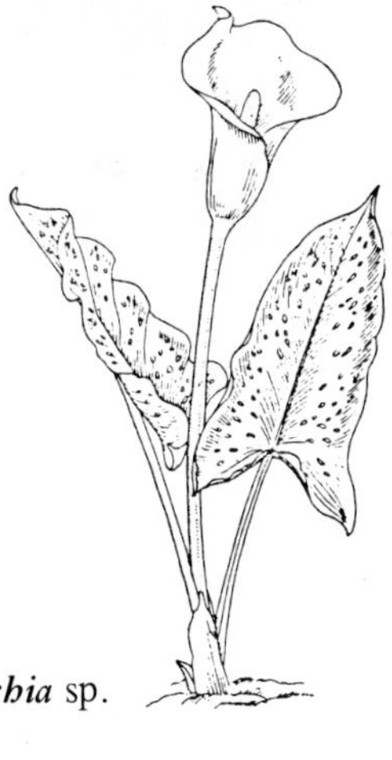

Zantedeschia sp.

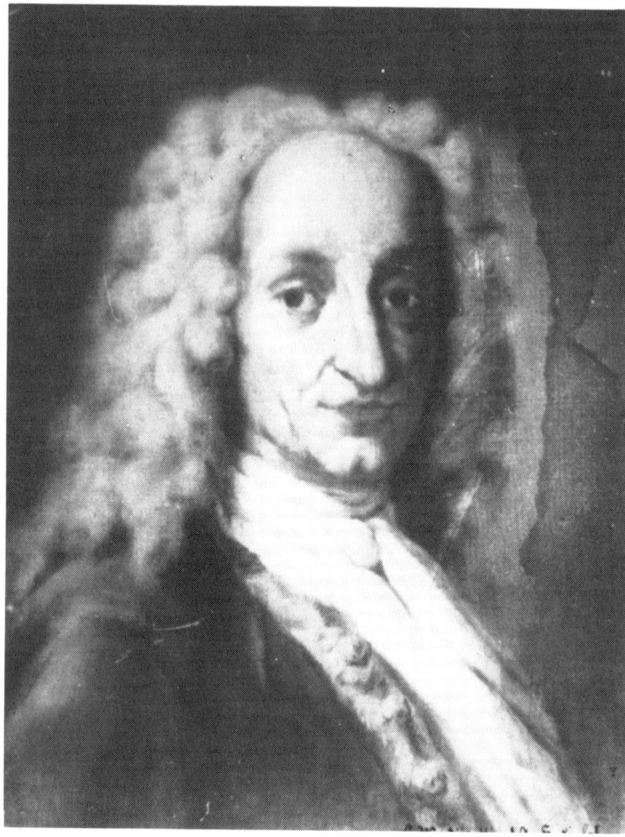

Dr GIOVANNI GIROLAMO ZANNICHELLI
(1662 – 1729)
Venetian doctor, pharmacist and botanist.

The Horned Pondweed, Zannichellia palustris, is a cosmopolitan species,; and although uncommon in Australia is found near Newcastle and at Murray Bridge in South Australia.

Photo courtesy of The Hunt Institute for Botanical Documentation, Carnegie-Mellon University, Pittsburgh.

ZINN, Professor Johann Gottfried (1727–1759)

Major contributions to medicine, exploration, scholarship and civic life –

Physician, Botanist

Country of residence and civic and scientific contribution –

Germany (Schwabach, Göttingen)

Scientific Name –

Zinnia australis
(Sole endemic species in Australia, but another species *Z. peruviana* now naturalized)

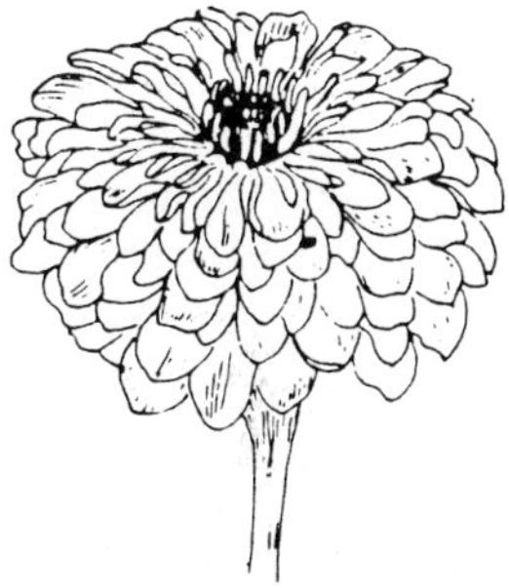

Zinnia sp.

ZORN, Dr Johannes (1739–1799)

Major contributions to medicine, exploration, scholarship and civic life –

Apothecary, Botanist, Senator

Country of residence and civic and scientific contribution –

Germany (Berlin, Kempten)

Scientific Name – Zornia spp.

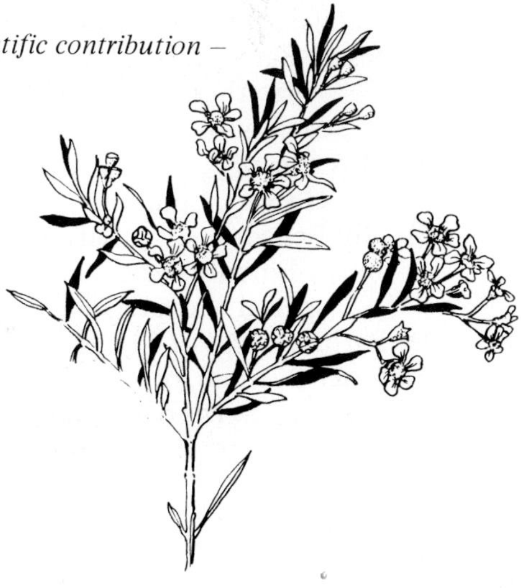

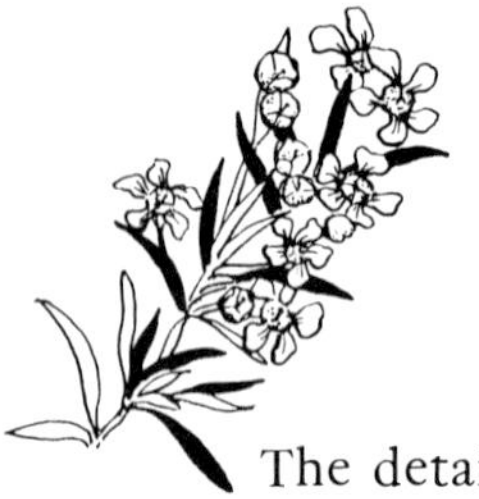

ACKNOWLEDGEMENTS

The detailed biographic research necessary for this work and its presentation as a medico-botanical cadaster could have been compiled only with the help of many friends. In particular, the author gratefully acknowledges the encouragement and support of –

Dr and Mrs Thomas Ackland, Consultant Surgeon, of Ivanhoe, Victoria;
Mr Robert Allen, skilled artist of The Queensland Museum, for his special generosity, and kindness;
Ms Julie Allum, Assistant Librarian, Royal College of Physicians, London;
Mr Barry Allwright, Photographer of Alice Springs, Northern Territory, for his generosity and encouragement;
Dr J.L. Anderton, Fellow & Secretary, Royal College of Physicians of Edinburgh;
Mr John Arnold, of The La Trobe Library, Melbourne;
Professor C.A. Atkins, Dept of Botany, University of Western Australia;
The Australian Systematic Botany Society, for their gracious permission to produce some of the line-drawings from *Flora of Central Australia*.

★

The late James Baines and his invaluable work *Australian Plant Genera*;
Professor Barry Baker of Dunedin, and Dean, Faculty of Anaesthetists, Royal Australasian College of Surgeons, Melbourne;
Mr M.A. Beasley, Botany Librarian, The British Museum of Natural History, London;
Mrs Ily Benedek, Librarian, Sydney Grammar School, Sydney;
Professor Emeritus Ragnar Berfenstam, of Uppsala, Sweden, for his special encouragement and help;
Dr Barbara Biggs of The Royal Botanic Gardens, Sydney;
Mr Peter Bostock, of The Queensland Herbarium, Brisbane;
Miss Dianne Byrne of The Oxley Library, State Library of Queensland, Brisbane, for her most gracious help and encouragement.

Mr Bob Campbell, Photographer, of the CSIRO, Melbourne;
Mr Charles Campbell, Priory Secretary, St John Ambulance Australia, of Canberra;
Mrs Martha Campbell (Mrs Martha Rutledge) of The Australian National University, Canberra;
Mrs Peggy Carter, of The Department of Child Health, Royal Children's Hospital, Brisbane, for her ongoing support and encouragement;
Mr Alan Clark, Assistant Librarian, The Royal Society, London;
Mr Alan Clark, Shoalhaven Historical Society, Nowra, N.S.W.;
Mr John Clarkson, Senior Botanist, Department of Primary Industries, Mareeba, Queensland;
Professor Trevor Clifford FLS, of The Department of Botany, University of Queensland, for much encouragement and help;
Mrs Cecily Close, Senior Archivist, University of Melbourne, Melbourne;
Professor Edward Cocking FRS, of The Department of Botany, The University of Nottingham, England;
Mrs Alison Corcoran, of The Department of Child Health, University of Queensland, Brisbane, for extensive help and ongoing support;
Ms Jeanette Covacevich, Senior Curator of The Queensland Museum, for extensive support and much encouragement;
Mrs Elwyn Coventry, of The Queensland Branch of the Australian Medical Association for her unstinting help;
Mr Des Cowley, of The La Trobe Library, State Library of Victoria;
Mr Geoffrey Cunningham of Killara, New South Wales, for encouragement, and his generosity in providing plates from *Plants of Western NSW* by G.M. Cunningham, W. Mulharn, P.L. Multhorpe, and J.A. Leigh;
Mrs Jo Currie, The Special Collections Librarian, Edinburgh University Library, Scotland, for much help, as on several previous occasions with other aspects of medical research;
Mr Raymond Curtis of North Tamborine, Queensland.

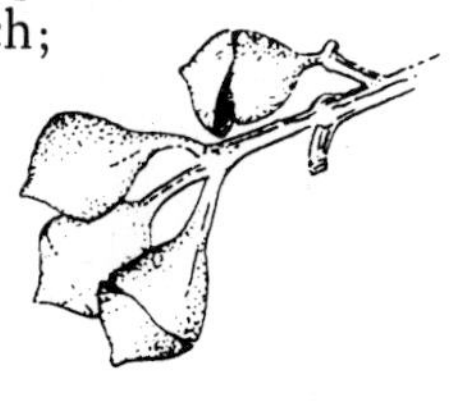

★

Professor John Dale, of Edinburgh;
Mr Geoffrey Davenport, Librarian to The Royal College of Physicians, London, for much encouragement on this as also on former occasions;
Mrs Gwenda Davis, of Port Macquarie, New South Wales;
Miss Allison Derrett, of Her Majesty's Royal Archives, Windsor, England;
Ms Frances Dimond, The Curator of The Photographic Collection, The Royal Archives, Windsor, England;
Mr Bob Dixon, Senior Botanical Adviser and Liaison Consultant of Kings Park and Botanic Gardens, Perth, for much ongoing help and support;
Mrs Ellen Donovan, of The Department of Child Health, University of Queensland, Brisbane, for much ongoing help and support;
Ms Gina Douglas, The Librarian of The Linnean Society of London;
Mr Ralph Dowling, Senior Botanist of The Queensland Herbarium, Brisbane, for much advice and encouragement;
Ms Christine Downer, Picture Librarian, State Library of Victoria;
Dr Sophie Ducker, Department of Botany, University of Melbourne;
Mrs Adi Dunlop, of Darwin, Northern Territory, for her gracious permission to reproduce several of her botanical drawings;

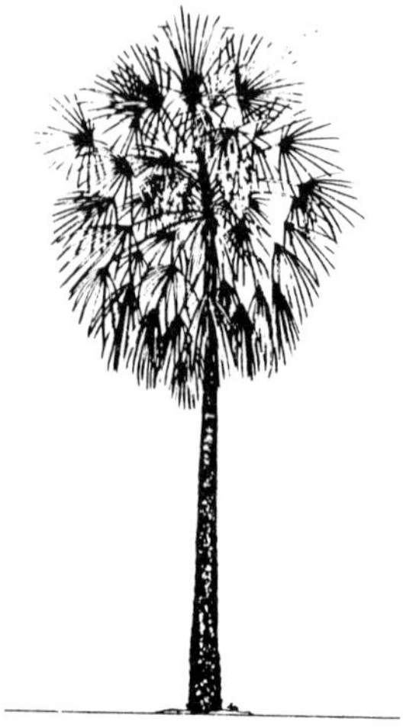

Dr Clyde Dunlop, of The Conservation Commission of the Northern Territory, Darwin;
Mr Ludwik Dutkiewicz of Adelaide for his fine botanical etchings.

★

Dr John Edmondson, National Museum and Galleries on Merseyside, Liverpool, U.K.;
M. Eppie Edwards of The National Library of Jamaica, Jamaica;
Mrs Sheila Edwards, Librarian, The Royal Society, London.

Mr Murray Fagg, Chief Information Officer of The Australian National Botanic Gardens, Canberra, and Consultant Photographer, for much help and encouragement, and for the provision of photographic slides from his personal collection;

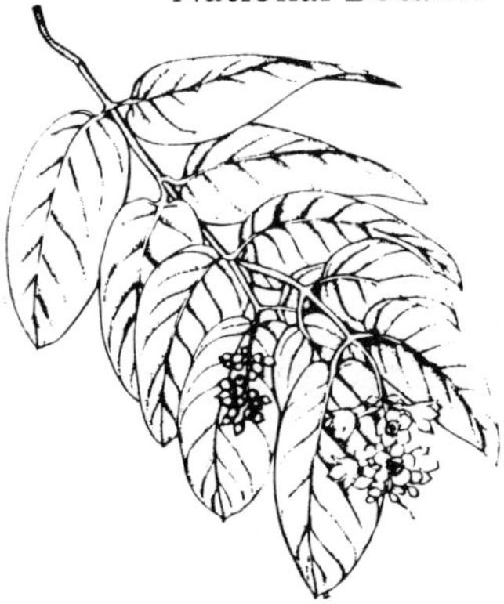

Mrs Joan Ferguson, Librarian, The Royal College of Physicians, Edinburgh, Scotland;

Miss Amelia Field DStJ of St John Ambulance Australia, in Melbourne;

Mr S.M.D. FitzGerald, Chief Librarian, Royal Botanic Gardens, Kew, Surrey;

Mrs Betty Foord, State Library of Victoria, Melbourne;

Dr J. Franklin, National Portrait Gallery, Lewisham, London;

Mr Bruce Fuhrer, of The Department of Botany and Zoology, Monash University, Melbourne, for much help and encouragement, and the provision of photographic slides from his personal collection.

★

Dr Christopher Gardner-Thorpe, Consultant Neurologist, of Devon, U.K., for much help and warm encouragement;

Dr Felix Garmendia, Real Jardin Botanico, Madrid, Spain;

Dr Alex George, Bureau of Flora and Fauna, Canberra;

Dr Lionel Gilbert of Armidale, N.S.W., for his spontaneous help and collaboration in the area of several biographic studies;

Dr Piero Giorgi, Department of Anatomy, University of Queensland;

The Government Printer, Queensland (for kind permission to reproduce certain line drawings from *Weeds of Queensland* by H.E. Kleinschmidt and Dr Robert Johnson);

Mrs Elizabeth Graham, Information Officer, The Royal Society, London;

Mr Bruce Gray, Botanist and Photographer of Atherton, North Queensland, for help with photographic slides from his personal collection;

Mr Ted Gregory of Mount Tamborine, Queensland, for much encouragement and help with detailed slides from his personal photographic collections of Australian native orchids;
Professor Kees Grooss, Curator of the Museum Boerhaave, Leiden, Holland;
Dr Desmond Gurry, of The Department of Child Health, University of Western Australia, Perth, for his spontaneous and infectious encouragement, and much trouble in helping with biographic and other details relating to this work;
Dr Gordon Guymer, of The Queensland Herbarium, Brisbane, for his time, and tolerant instruction;
Professor Richard Gye, former Dean of the Faculty of Medicine, University of Sydney, Sydney.

★

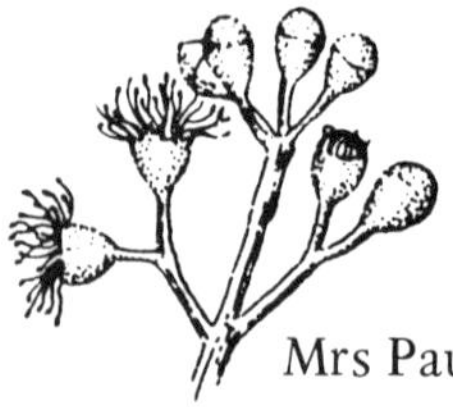

Mr Norman Hall, Consultant Botanist and eucalypt specialist of Castle Hill, Sydney;
Mr Victor Halin, of the Gold Coast, Queensland;
Mrs Pauline Hanna, of The Bath Historical Association, Bath, U.K., for her warm and unstinting help;
Dr William Hanna, Surgeon, of Bendigo, Victoria;
Mr Ron Hastings, The Executive Director of The Australian Medical Association [Victorian Branch], Melbourne, for his considerable expenditure of time, and much encouragement;
Miss Brenda Heagney, The Librarian, The Royal Australasian College of Physicians, Sydney, for her ongoing warm encouragement and much help;
Dr Elwyn and Dr Mervyn Hegarty of Indooroopilly, Brisbane, for their longstanding personal friendship, and much help and encouragement;
Dr Helen Hewson, Bureau of Flora and Fauna, Canberra;
Mr Chris Hill, of The Department of Palaeontology, The British Museum of Natural History, London, for his detailed and spontaneous help and advice;
Miss Joan Hoare of the Professional Typesetting Services, University of Queensland, Brisbane, for ongoing help with publication;

Dr Athel Hockey of Perth;
Dr Alison Hogg of Ringwood, Victoria;
Ms Joan Horsley, National Maritime Museum, Greenwich, London;
Ms Sheila Houghton, The Field Naturalists Club of Victoria, Melbourne, for considerable research into archival details and much help;
The Hunt Institute for Botanical Documentation (The Carnegie Mellon University), Pittsburgh, U.S.A., for considerable help, and much encouragement spontaneously proferred.

★

Dr Surrey Jacobs, of The Royal Botanic Gardens, Sydney;
Mr Robert Jago of Manunda, North Queensland, for his gracious generosity in providing advice and photographic slides from his personal photographic collection of North Queensland species;
Dr John Jessop for help and encouragement, and also for kind permission to reproduce several line drawings from *Flora of Central Australia*;
Dr Laurie Jessup, Botanist, of The Queensland Herbarium, Brisbane;
M. Asa Johansson, of the Uppsala Turist and Kongress AB, Uppsala, Sweden;
Dr Robert Johnson, The Director of The Queensland Herbarium, Brisbane, for much personal help, and also for kind permission to reproduce some line drawings from his publication (with Dr Harry Kleinschmidt) from their work *Weeds of Queensland*;
Ms Nicolaine Jordan and Mr Lester Markwell of Coochiemudlo Island, Queensland, for their warm ongoing friendship and much encouragement;
Mr Graham and Mrs Esther Jurott, Medical Photographers, Faculty of Medicine, University of Queensland, Brisbane.

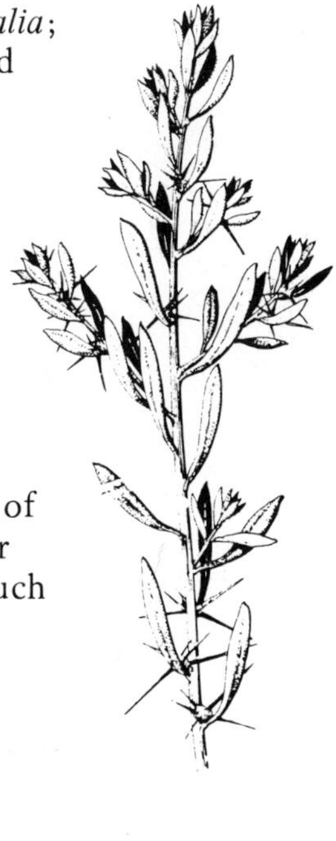

Professor C. Kalkman, Rijksherbarium, Leiden, The Netherlands;
Dr M.G. Kanowski, Department of Classics and Ancient History, University of Queensland;
Ms Anita Karg, of The Hunt Institute for Botanical Documentation, (Carnegie Mellon University), Pittsburg, U.S.A., for her warm and spontaneous encouragement, and much help;
Mr Stan Kelly of Ararat, Victoria, for his generous provision of drawings from his personal collection, and for kind permission to reproduce several illustrations from both Volumes I and II of his encyclopaedic pictorial work *Eucalypts*;
Dr Kevin Kenneally, Senior Botanist, The Western Australian Herbarium, Perth, for much botanical advice and the provision of photographic slides from his personal collection;
Dr Geoffrey Kenny, The Department of Anatomy, University of Melbourne, Melbourne;
Ms Sheila Kruse, of Canberra, and the Kruse Family for biographic details.

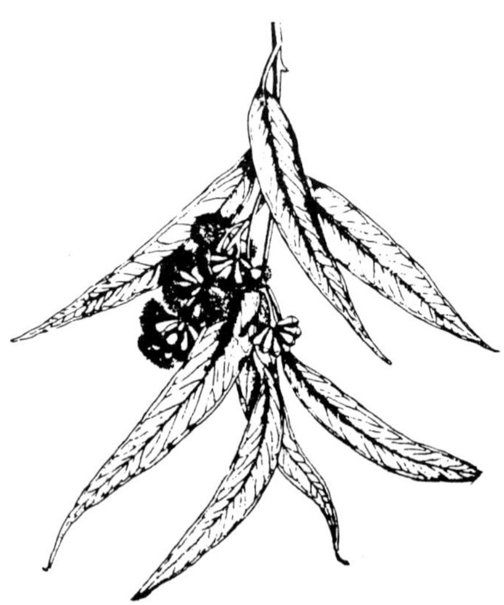

Mr and Mrs John Lahey of Indooroopilly, Brisbane, for advice and help, particularly in relation to orchid species;

Miss Henrietta Lang of Lismore, Victoria, for help with biographic details;

Mr Peter Latz, Botanist and Ecologist, of The Arid Zone Research Institute, The Conservation Commission of the Northern Territory at Alice Springs, for his time and warm encouragement, and the provision of specialised photographic material;

Mr Michael Lazarides, The National Herbarium, Canberra;

Mr Greg Leach, The Herbarium of the Northern Territory, Darwin;

Mrs Kathleen Lewellin, of Mentone, Victoria, for her warm help with biographic details;

Mr Allan ("Llew") Llewellyn of Eaglehawk, Victoria, for his warm and ongoing friendship, for much hospitality, and his advice and encouragement about cultivars bred in Australia;

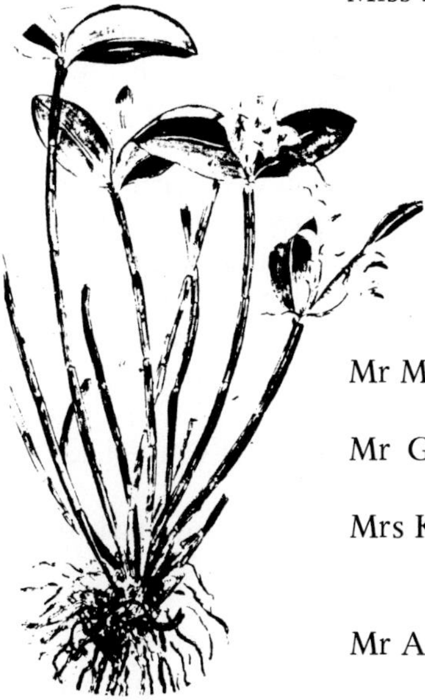

Dr James Love, Consultant Physician of Brisbane, for his help with biographic details;

Mr I.F. Lyle, The Librarian of The Royal College of Surgeons of London, U.K., for his help with specialised biographic details about early British surgeons;

Mrs Pat Lyndon, Librarian, Sydney Grammar School, Sydney.

★

Mr Stirling Macoboy, Horticulturist, Author and Photographer, of Sydney, for his most generous provision of photographic details, and for permission to quote from several of his reference works on garden horticulture;

Mrs Betty Malone of the Prahran Historical and Arts Society, Melbourne;
Mr Colin MacGregor of West Rosebud, Victoria;
Dr H.S. MacKee, Service Forestier, New Caledonia;
Mme. Agnes Marcetteau, Bibliotheque Municipale, Nantes, France;
Dr Elizabeth Marks, Queensland Institute of Medical Research, Brisbane;
Mrs Joan Martin, Brownless Library, University of Melbourne;
Mr and Mrs Stewart McCracken of Caloundra, Queensland;
Mr William Fancourt McDonald, The Queensland Herbarium, Brisbane;
Ms Judith McKay, Senior Curator of The Queensland Museum, Brisbane, for her warm encouragement and help with water-colour illustrations from the Ellis Rowan Collection of The Queensland Museum;
Mr Ross McKinnon, Curator, The Botanic Gardens, Mt Coot-tha, Brisbane;
Dr Rod McLeod AO,RFD,ED, President, The Queensland Maritime Museum;
Ms Pamela McLure, Royal Women's Hospital, Melbourne;
Mr Frank McMahon of Canberra, for his gracious permission to include some examples from his poetry which so captures the historical feeling of early local community life in Australia;
Ms Kristie McRobert, State Library of Victoria, Melbourne;
Mrs Enid Meldrum, Librarian, The Alfred Hospital, Melbourne;
Mr R.A. Mills, Head, Library Information Services, University of Oxford, England;
Professor Bob Milns, Department of Classics & Ancient History, University of Queensland;
Dr Ann Mitchell, Historian, of Melbourne;
The Mitchell Library, State Library of New South Wales – for kind permission to reproduce the figure of *Amyema gaudichaudii* by Helena Scott, from the Library's Collection;
Dr Geoffrey Monteith, The Queensland Museum, Brisbane;
Dr Brian Morley, Botanic Gardens, of Adelaide;
Mr Doug Moss of The Gap, Brisbane.

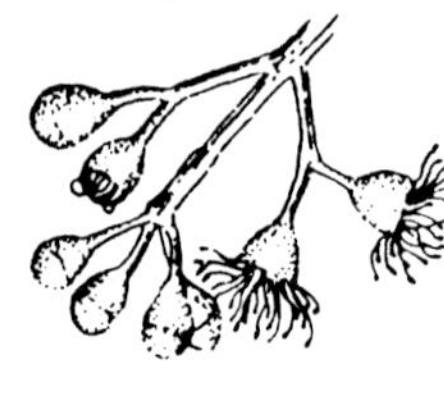

The National Portrait Gallery, London, for permission to reproduce photographs and portraits in the British National Collection;

Mr Neville Naumann, Dahlia Specialist of Bracken Ridge, Brisbane;

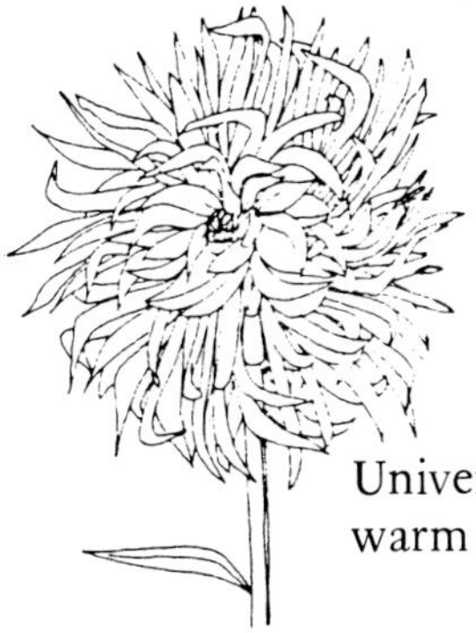

Mrs Jan and Mr Hugh Nicholson of "Tristania" Rainforest Nursery of Lismore, New South Wales, for much encouragement and for their most gracious and generous provision of photographs and rainforest plants and trees from their personal collection;

Dr James Nixon, Department of Child Health, University of Queensland, Brisbane, for his continued warm friendship and ongoing support.

★

Dr Peter Oelrichs, The Animal Research Institute, Brisbane;

Mr Brenden O'Keefe, Medical Historian, War Memorial, Canberra;

Ms Jane Oliver, Librarian, The Royal Australasian College of Surgeons, Melbourne;

Ms Kate O'Mara, Librarian, Town Hall, South Melbourne.

★

Mrs Lynne Packer, Department of Child Health, University of Queensland, for her ongoing warm encouragement and good humour in the preparation of this manuscript;

Mrs Susan Patrick, The West Australian Herbarium, Perth;

Dr Robert Pearce, Consultant Plastic and Reconstructive Surgeon, of Perth, for much hospitality and warm friendship and encouragement;

Mr Les Pedley, The Queensland Herbarium, Brisbane;

Ms Barbara Perry and Ms Esther Robinson, Pictorial Librarians, National Library of Australia, Canberra;

Mr Andrew Petrie, Chief Pharmaceutical Consultant of The State Health Department, Queensland, for warm friendship and help with biographic details;

Mr J.L. Priestly, Secretary, National Rose Society of Australia;

Mrs Janet Pullen, Dept of Child Health, University of Queensland, Brisbane.

The Queensland Herbarium and staff for the access to resources and much help;
The Queensland Museum, Brisbane, for the provision of much help, and their gracious permission to reproduce several photographs from the Museum's Collection.

★

Mr Paul Ramsden, The Graphics Unit, The Queensland Museum, Brisbane, for his skilled artistry, encouragement and warm advice;
Ms Thekla Reichstein, The Botanic Gardens of Adelaide, Adelaide;
Ms Angela Renfrey, Botany Department, University of Adelaide;
Professor M.D. Rickard of the CSIRO, Melbourne;
Professor William Ritchie, Professor of Greek, University of Sydney, Sydney;
Dr Barbara Robertson of Shepparton, Victoria;
The Royal Botanic Gardens, Kew, Surrey, U.K.;
Mr David Ruston of Renmark, South Australia.

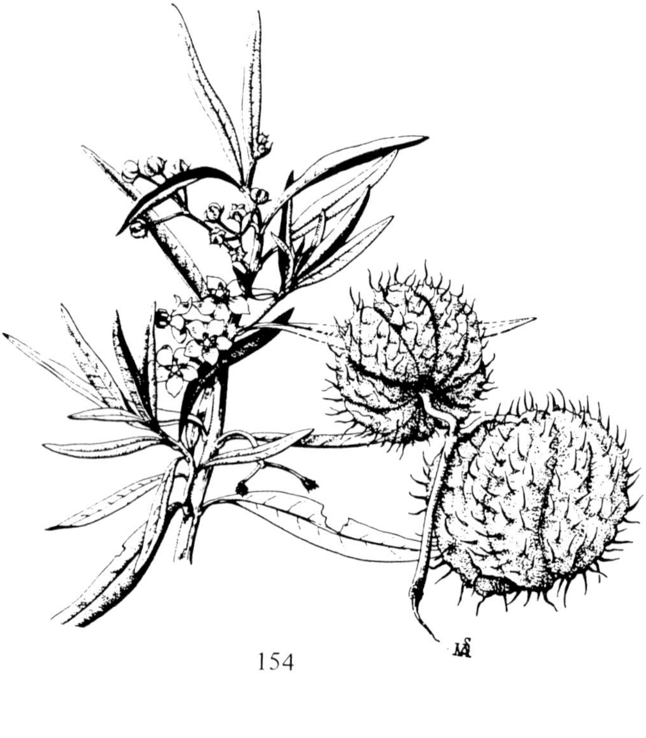

Ms Margaret Saul, formerly the Botanical Illustrator, The Queensland Herbarium, Brisbane;
Mr Charles Scandrett and Staff, Merino Lithographics, Moorooka, Brisbane;
Dr Heinrich Schaupp, Consultant ENT Surgeon of Everton Park, Brisbane, for much help with translation of documents and biographic accounts;
Dr Louise Schofield, Department of Greek and Roman Antiquities, The British Museum, London;
Ms Jenny Scott of The Geography Department, University of Tasmania, Hobart;
Dr Rodney Seppelt of The Department of Sciences, The Australian Antarctic Division, Hobart, Tasmania, for his spontaneous and warm help and botanical advice;
Mr Francis Sharr, whose work *Western Australian Plant Names and Their Meanings*, was a most helpful reference source in this undertaking;
Ms Julia Sheppard, The Wellcome Institute, London;
Dr P.S. Short, The National Herbarium of Victoria, Melbourne;
Dr Eric Sims AM, Consultant Paediatrician of Adelaide, South Australia, for his warm encouragement and personal friendship;
Mrs Doris Sinkora, The National Herbarium of Victoria, Melbourne, for much detailed help in the area of biographic research;
Dr Ron Southcott of Mitcham, Adelaide;
Mr Kenneth Smith, Archivist, University of Sydney, Sydney;
Mr Will Smith, Botanical Illustrator, The Queensland Herbarium, Brisbane;
Mr Walter Strive, State Library of Victoria, Melbourne;
Ms Valerie Swane, for encouragement, and permission to quote from several of her horticultural works;
Dr David Symon, The Botanic Gardens of Adelaide, Adelaide, South Australia.

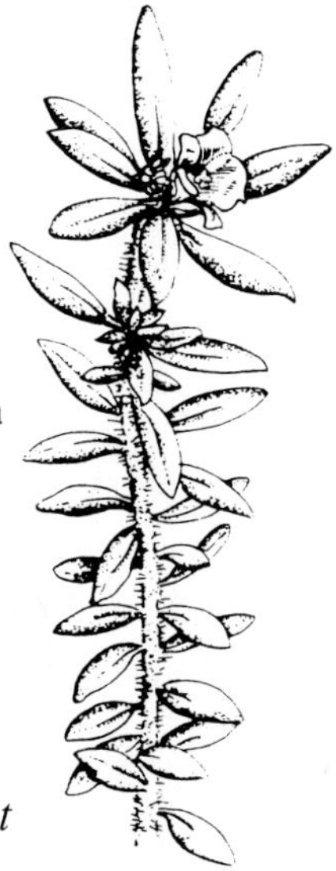

★

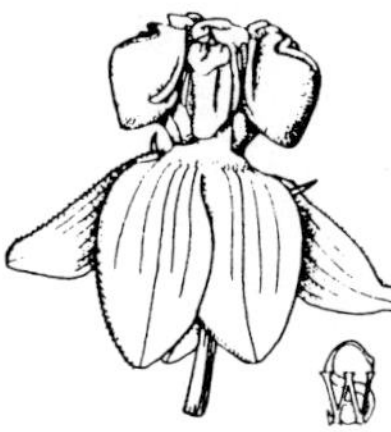

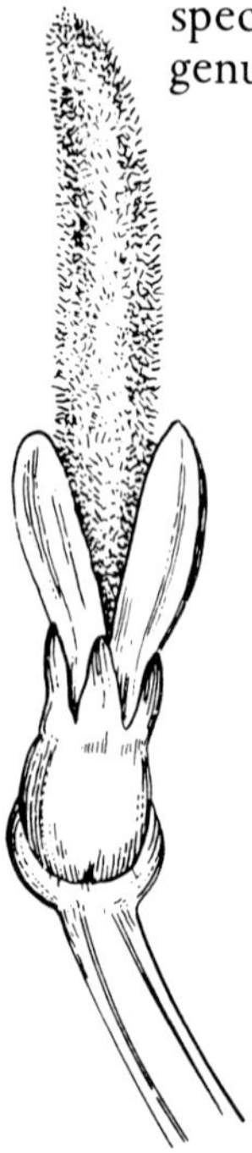

Dr Lorraine Tan (née Durrington) of Buderim, Queensland, for specific help in relation to the newly described tribe and genus of plants which bears her name;

Ms Kay Thomas of Brisbane, for help with Danish translations;

Mrs Merle Thompson, The Blue Mountains Group of the Society for Growing Australian Plants, for her enthusiastic help, photography, and the collection of several species which form the text of this work;

Ms Prue Timpson-Wearne, of Hammersley Iron Pty Ltd, Dampier, West Australia, for her warm help and encouragement, and her generosity in providing several slides from her personal photographic collection;

Mrs Ursula Tokle (née Maunsell) of The Royal Society, London, for her warm personal friendship and ongoing encouragement.

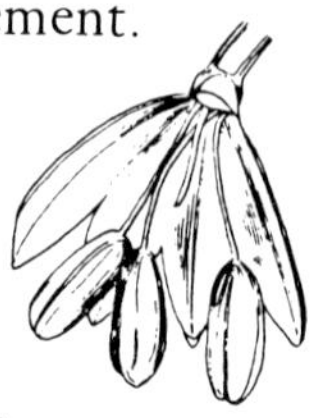

★

The Victorian College of Pharmacy, Melbourne, Victoria.

★

Professor Dr G. Wagenitz of Göttingen, West Germany;

Miss J. Ward, Librarian, Royal Botanic Gardens, Kew, Surrey, U.K.;

Docteur Christian Warolin, Secrétaire Général de la Société d'Histoire de la Pharmacie, Paris;

Dr Colin Waterford of The Division of Entomology, CSIRO, Canberra, for his help with botanical and biographic details relating to early wheat varieties in Australia;

The Western Australian Wildflower Society (Inc.) and its secretary, Ms Denise Marchant, of Perth;

Dr Mary White, Consultant Palaeobotanist, of Sydney, for her detailed advice in the area of the taxonomy of fossil plants in Australia, for the provision of several slides from her personal collection, and for permission to quote from her book *The Greening of Gondwana*;

Dr William Wilkie, Psychiatrist, of Brisbane;

Dr Lesley Williams, Department of Anatomy, University of Queensland, Brisbane;

Mr Morris Williams, Librarian, Victorian College of Pharmacy, Melbourne, for much help with biographical details relating to several early Australian pharmacists;

Mrs Jan Wilson, Photographic Curator of The Australian National Botanic Gardens, Canberra, for much warm encouragement;

Dr Karen Wilson, Royal Botanic Gardens, Sydney, and formerly the Australian Liaison Officer, The Royal Botanic Gardens, Kew, London;

Dr R. Wright, Librarian, Parliament House, Melbourne;

Dr Paul Wycherley OBE, The Director, King's Park and Botanic Gardens, Perth, for his warm hospitality and encouragement.

The publication of this work was possible especially because of the dedication of Mrs Alison Corcoran and Mrs Peggy Carter of the Department of Child Health, Royal Children's Hospital in Brisbane, to whom the author pays special tribute.

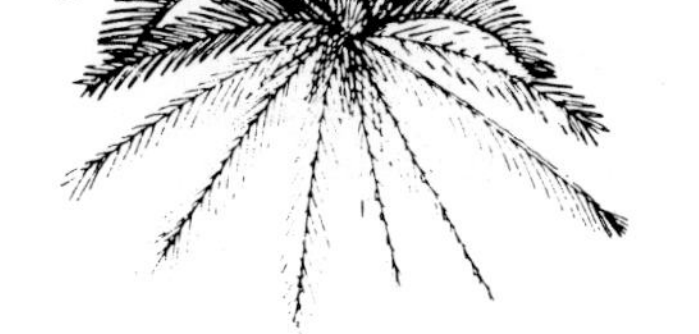

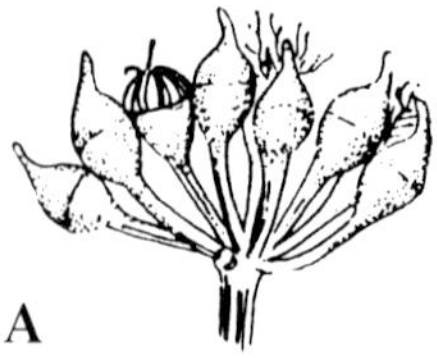

INDEX

A (contd)

B

B (contd)

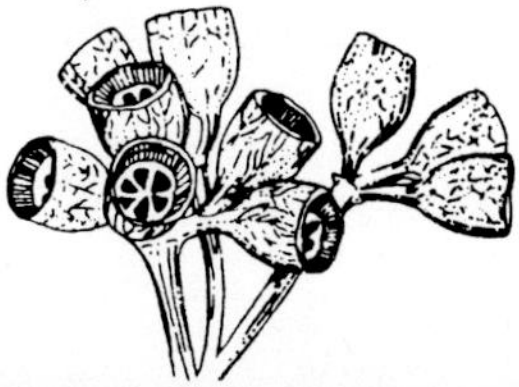

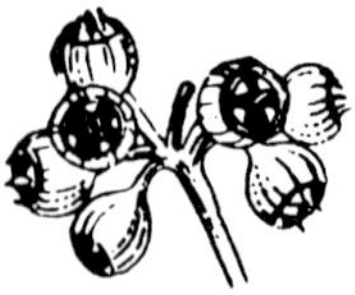

Index

B (contd)

B (contd)

C

C (contd)

C (contd)

D

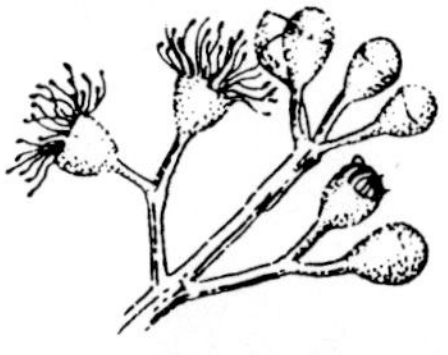

D (contd)

E

E (contd)

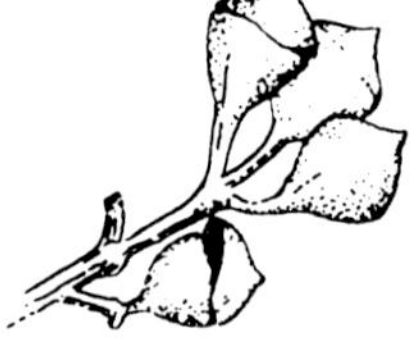

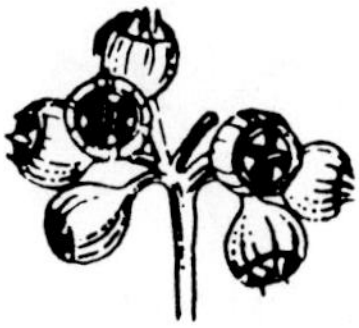

F

G

G (contd)

H

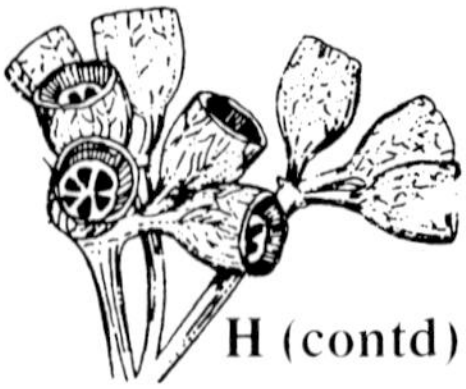

H (contd)

I

J

K

L

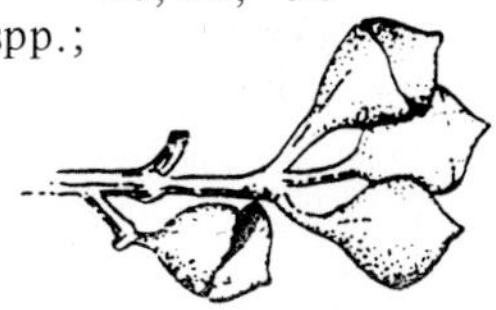

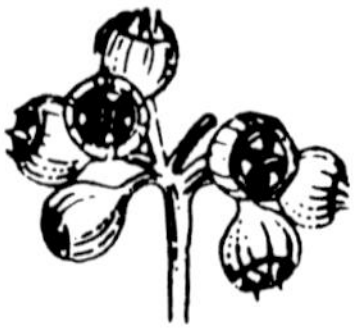

Index

P (contd)

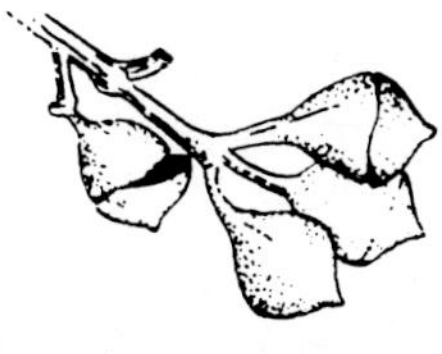

Q

R

S

S (contd)

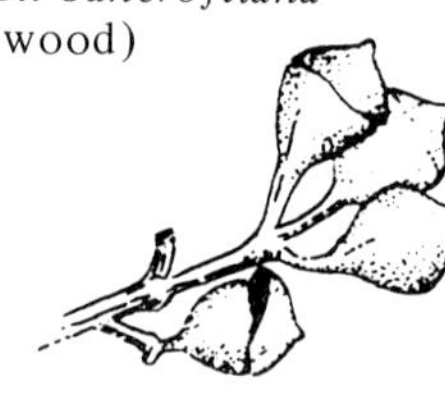

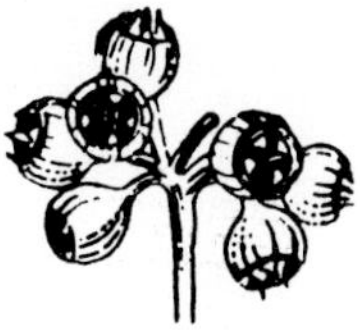

W (contd)

W (contd)

X

Y

Z

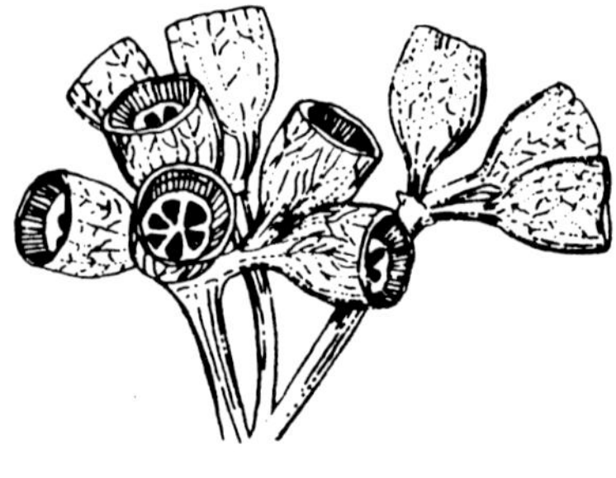

BACK COVER

The back cover of this medico-botanical cadaster illustrates six doctor-botanists whose names are perpetuated in Australian native plants. They span four centuries of human endeavour and research into the living world that blooms around us.

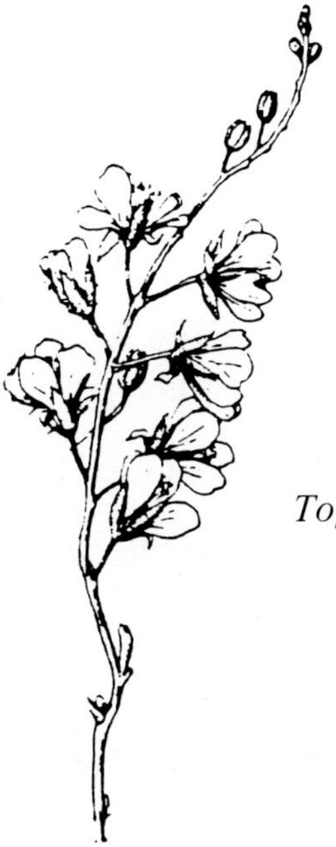

Top Left:

Professor Andrea Caesalpino (1519–1603), Professor of Medicine at Pisa (from 1555) and at Rome (from 1952). One of the founders of modern scientific botany, he was one of the first to develop a rational system of plant classification. The genus *Caesalpinia* and the Family *Caesalpiniaceae* commemorate his name.

Top Right:

Dr James Rudall (1828–1907) – medical practitioner, ophthalmologist and ENT surgeon of Melbourne, Australia. He had served as a naval surgeon and had travelled to Arctic regions before emigrating to Australia. He was also a skilled musician. The Australian plant, *Myriocephalus rudallii* honours him.

Centre Left:

Dr Richard Sanders Rogers (1862–1942) – Consultant physician of Adelaide, Australia. A Foundation Fellow of the Royal Australasian College of Physicians (in 1938) and Member of the Medical Board of South Australia (1911–1940), he was one of the foremost authorities on Australian orchids; and was elected a Fellow of the Linnean Society in 1924. The greenhood orchid, *Pterostylis rogersii*, commemorates his life and works.

Back Cover

Centre Right:

Surgeon Robert Brown (1773–1858) – Father of Australian Botany. A Scottish military surgeon who served originally with the Fifeshire Fencibles, he came to Australia as surgeon and botanist with Matthew Flinders. He circumnavigated Australia with Flinders in 1802–1803 and collected and named thousands of new species of plants. On his return to London he worked as a botanist and librarian to Sir Joseph Banks. The genera *Brunonia* and *Brunoniella*, and dozens of species which bear his name immortalize his contributions to natural history.

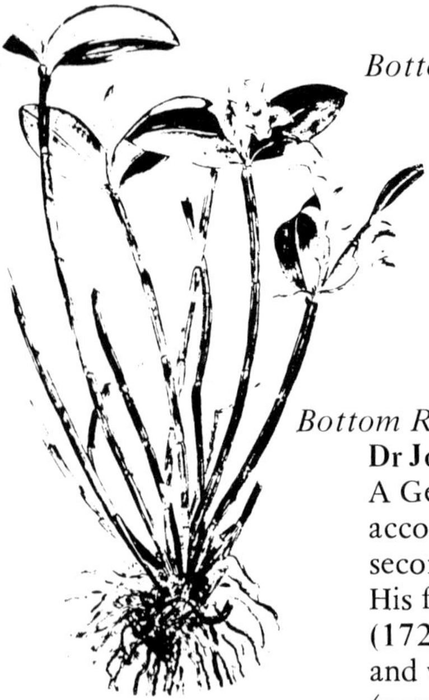

Bottom Left:

Dr Hugo Flecker (1884–1957) – General Practitioner and Radiologist of Cairns, Queensland. An eminent botanist and zoologist, the beautiful orchid of Mt Bartle Frere, *Dendrobium fleckeri*, was named in his honour.

Bottom Right:

Dr Johann Georg Adam Forster (1754–1794). A German-born doctor and naturalist, he accompanied Captain James Cook on his second Australian voyage, on HMS *Resolution.* His father, **Dr Johann Reinhold Forster (1729–1798)** was his patron and mentor, and was with him on the voyage. Johann (portrayed here in an engraving by courtesy of the Hunt Institute for Botanical Documentation) wrote "A Voyage around the World in His Britannic Majesty's Ship, *Resolution*" which was published in 1777.